Clinical Assessment and Monitoring in Children

Diana Fergusson
RGON (NZ), RSCN, MNS, PG Dip HPE, BN,
Int Care Cert, Paed and NN Int Care Cert
Lecturer Practitioner
PICU
Oxford Radcliffe NHS Hospital Trust
Oxford

Contributor
Lorrie Lawton
Lecturer Practitioner
Emergency Department
Oxford Radcliffe NHS Hospital Trust
Oxford

Debbie Marth

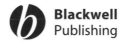

D1390493

Blackwell
Publishing

Blackwell Publishing editorial offices:
Blackwell Publishing Ltd, 9600 Garsington Road, Oxford OX4 2DQ, UK
Tel: +44 (0)1865 776868
Blackwell Publishing Inc., 350 Main Street, Malden, MA 02148-5020, USA
Tel: +1 781 388 8250
Blackwell Publishing Asia Pty Ltd, 550 Swanston Street, Carlton, Victoria 3053, Australia
Tel: +61 (0)3 8359 1011

First published 2008 by Blackwell Publishing Ltd

ISBN: 978-1-4051-3338-8

Library of Congress Cataloging-in-Publication Data

Fergusson, Diana.
Clinical assessment and monitoring in children / Diana Fergusson.
p. ; cm. – (Essential clinical skills for nurses)
Includes bibliographical references and index.
ISBN-13: 978-1-4051-3338-8 (pbk.:alk. paper)
ISBN-10: 1-4051-3338-4 (pbk.:alk. paper)   1. Pediatric nursing.   2. Nursing assessment.   3. Pediatric intensive care.   I. Title.   II. Series.
[DNLM: 1. Child.   2. Nursing Assessment–methods.   3. Nursing Care–methods.   4. Pediatric Nursing–methods. WY 100.4 F352c 2008]
RJ245.F45 2008
618.92'00231–dc22
2007037123

A catalogue record for this title is available from the British Library

Set in 9 on 11pt Palatino by SNP Best-set Typesetter Ltd., Hong Kong
Printed and bound in Singapore by Utopia Press Pte Ltd

The publisher's policy is to use permanent paper from mills that operate a sustainable forestry policy, and which has been manufactured from pulp processed using acid-free and elementary chlorine-free practices. Furthermore, the publisher ensures that the text paper and cover board used have met acceptable environmental accreditation standards.

For further information on Blackwell Publishing, visit our website:
www.blackwellpublishing.com

Contents

Preface   iv

Acknowledgements   v

1   Introduction   1

2   Respiratory Assessment   13

3   Respiratory Monitoring   42

4   Cardiovascular Assessment   79

5   Cardiovascular Monitoring and
    Haemodynamics   103

6   Neurological Assessment   134

7   Acute Neurological Assessment and
    Monitoring   166

8   The Gastro-intestinal System and Abdomen   191

9   Nutrition   204

10 Fluid and Electrolytes   231

11 The Head and Neck   250

12 The Musculoskeletal System   280

13 Temperature Monitoring   296

14 Comfort and Hygiene   311

Index   339

Preface

Welcome to the first edition of *Clinical Assessment and Monitoring in Children*. Children are no longer considered as little adults; their physiology and response to illness is very different to adults and therefore they need a different approach with regard to assessment and monitoring.

Health care practitioners require a range of examination techniques to choose from depending on the different age groups and clinical presentations. This book provides the reader with a comprehensive range of approaches. I hope that all those caring for children will find it a valuable resource.

Diana Fergusson

Acknowledgements

The author is grateful to:

- Neila Chrisp, Head Nurse, PICU, John Radcliffe Hospital, for her generous support to undertake this publication.
- Clare Burnett, Clinical Nurse Specialist, Gastro-enterology, for her assistance with Chapter 9.
- Jackie Campbell, Clinical Nurse Specialist, Neurology, John Radcliffe Hospital, for her assistance with Chapter 7.
- Staff and students of PICU, John Radcliffe Hospital, for their valuable feedback.
- Teresa Finlay, Senior Lecturer, Oxford Brookes University, for her advice and encouragement.
- Jeff Churcher, my husband, for his immense support and his help in providing the illustrations.

Introduction

1

INTRODUCTION

This book is designed for heath care practitioners learning to care for sick children. All children routinely have assessment and monitoring performed on them as part of their overall care. Assessment is the collection of data including subjective (what the child/family says) and objective (what the health care practitioner finds with the techniques of inspection, palpation, percussion and auscultation). Monitoring is the recording of specific data, often using a device.

LEARNING OBJECTIVES

By the end of this chapter the reader will be able to:

❏ Understand the key components in undertaking a comprehensive health history.
❏ Introduce some concepts of assessment and principles of examination techniques in different child age groups.

CHILD AGES

Childhood is a time of growth and development into adulthood and therefore children are not small adults and should not be considered as such. Physiologically, adolescence approaches adulthood and young people may be treated medically within an adult framework. Table 1.1 outlines the terms clarifying different age groups (Wong 1995; Gill & O'Brien 2002).

Young children are unable to articulate clearly their problems and may demonstrate unwellness in other ways. Look for the child who is:

• quiet (abnormally so);
• not eating or refusing food (even when it is a favourite);

- lying down or adopting a position that is most comfortable to him or her.

HISTORY-TAKING

History-taking aims to achieve a complete picture of the child's health status (Jarvis 2003).

Identifying data

Data must adhere to local policy and legal requirements, including:

- name
- parents' details
- address and phone number
- date of birth
- school attended
- ethnicity

Chief complaint and history of presenting illness

Most information about the unwell child will come from the history. Often the mother or the primary carer is the key person to verbalise concerns. The primary carer will know the child best of all and will know when something is not quite right. Ask them what they think is wrong; their intuition is usually good. It is important to document exactly what the child/carer states is wrong with the child as misinterpretation of what has been said can mislead the assessment and management of the problem.

Table 1.1 Classification of age groups.

Classification	Age ranges
Newborn/neonate	0–28 days
Infant	1–12 months
Toddler	1–3 years
Pre-schooler	3–5 years
School age	5–18 years
Early adolescent	10–14 years
Late adolescent	15–18 years

Table 1.2 OLDCART: a model of history taking.

Key issues	Example questions
O = onset	When did it start?
L = location	Where is it (point to it)? Does it go anywhere? Is it superficial or deep?
D = duration	How long does it last? How often does it come?
C = characteristics	What effects does it have on the child (stops him or her playing, eating)? Is it sharp, dull, aching, throbbing, shooting, burning? How strong is it? Is it constant or intermittent? What brings it on? Does it occur in a specific environment or with specific activities or a particular emotional state?
A = associated symptoms	Are there any other symptoms?
R = relieving/aggravating symptoms	What makes it better? What makes it worse?
T = treatments	What have you done to treat it?

Establishing a good relationship, including optimal listening skills, is therefore most important. Clarify what is meant by terms that are used to describe a sign or symptom. Let the child/parent/caregiver talk about concerns, then use a model or framework to capture specific information on the history of present illness. Table 1.2 outlines one model, and taking a history of pain is used as an example (Bickley 2003). Check that you:

- ask only one question at a time;
- refrain from use of jargon;
- are not judgmental;
- are not using vague terms.

Past medical history
Pregnancy and birth details are particularly important for the child who is less than 2 years of age or who has any neurological or developmental problems (Engel 1997). Ask about:

(1) Pregnancies
- number of pregnancies and the outcome of these;
- the pregnancy of this child:
  - nausea and vomiting
  - vaginal bleeding
  - unusual or unexplained weight gain
  - weight loss
  - blood pressure
  - oedema
  - accidents
  - results of any fetal heart scan
  - infections
  - drug-taking: prescribed, over-the-counter and recreational (known teratogens include phenytoin, warfarin, lithium, carbamazepine, trimethodione, sodium valproate) (Archer & Birch 1998)
  - alcohol use
  - maternal diabetes (increased risk of congenital heart disease (CHD)
  - other maternal medical history (increased risk of CHD with phenylketonuria, systemic lupus erythematosus)
  - rubella in first trimester (known teratogen)
  - age of mother at birth (over 40 years involves increased risk of genetic disorders, e.g. Trisomy 21).

(2) Birth
- spontaneous or induced labour;
- normal vaginal delivery, vertex, breech or caesarean section delivery;
- term or premature;
- APGAR – see Table 1.3 (a tool used at 1 minute and 5 minutes after birth) (Farrell & Sittlington 2003);
- any problems at birth and the outcomes of these;
- birth weight;
- congenital infections;
- respiratory difficulty and the outcome of this.

(3) Neonatal period: if any problems occurred and what the outcome was:
- jaundice
- colic

Table 1.3 APGAR scores.

Measure	Score 0	Score 1	Score 2
Appearance (colour)	Pale or blue	Centrally pink, peripherally blue	Pink
Pulse (heart rate)	Zero	<100	>100
Grimace (response to stimuli, e.g. suctioning of pharynx)	No response	Grimace	Cry
Active (muscle tone)	Limp	Some flexion in extremities	Good flexion
Respirations	Zero	Slow and irregular, weak cry	Normal, good cry

- breathing difficulties
- feeding problems
- seizures
- mother's health.

(4) Feeding (see Chapter 9).

(5) Growth and development (see Chapter 6).

Previous illnesses, operations or injuries

- Childhood illnesses (including measles, mumps, chicken pox) and any recent exposure to illness, foreign travel.
- Accidents and injuries; the extent of injuries, the treatment and any complications.
- Serious illnesses, admissions to hospital/operations; the extent of injuries, the treatment and any complications, the child's reaction to being in hospital.
- Minor illnesses.
- Chronic illnesses; onset, treatment and any complications.

Immunisations

- Specific details of schedule.

Allergies

- Include medications, food and pollen and what symptoms may be suffered.

Medications

- All over-the-counter, prescribed and complementary therapy.
- The use of tobacco, social drugs and/or alcohol.

Family history

- Draw a genogram (also known as a family tree). Figure 1.1 shows an example.

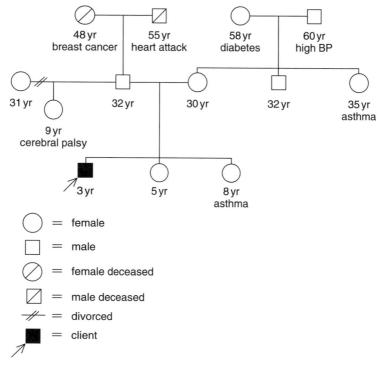

Fig. 1.1 A genogram.

- Include age and cause of deaths in the family.
- Establish who is the family of this child and any support systems, e.g. neighbour, friend, grandparents.
- Exposure to smoking.
- Any history in the family similar to the symptoms of the child.
- Hypertension, vascular disease (cardiac, cerebral, peripheral), kidney problems, diabetes mellitus, cancer, blood disorders, arthritis, allergies, mental illness, seizures, learning difficulties.
- Genetic or congenital disorders: include enquiry into any dysmorphism to see if there are any congenital underlying causes.

Psychosocial history
- Single or married/de facto relationship.
- Parent employment.
- Housing (Goldbloom 1997).
- Social care assistance.
- Any child protection issues.

Review of systems
This helps to evaluate previous and current status of the body systems and checks that nothing has been missed so far. It may be more useful to write that a symptom is either present or absent rather than labelling a system as 'negative'. In this scenario, it is unclear exactly what has been assessed. Check with the carer/child about any problems they have experienced with each of the systems, including (see subsequent chapters for further details):

- general health: weight (loss, increase), fatigue, general wellness
- skin: eczema
- head and neck: head, eyes, ears, nose, mouth, throat, neck
- breasts
- respiratory: coughs, colds
- cardiovascular: heart disease
- gastro-intestinal: diarrhoea, vomiting

- renal
- genital
- musculoskeletal: fractures
- neurological: any loss of consciousness
- haematological: bleeding
- endocrine: diabetes
- psychiatric

PHYSICAL EXAMINATION

Objective data can be obtained with the use of physical examination techniques. These are fully described for each system in subsequent chapters. Some techniques are considered advanced and will be noted as such. Children have the right to privacy and maintenance of dignity during examination. Although the chapters provide a systematic approach to examination, the health care practitioner needs to be opportunistic in gathering objective data. The following techniques are the cornerstone of comprehensive physical examination and are usually undertaken in the following order. However, flexibility is essential in examining children; taking opportunities and going from least disturbing to most disturbing may provide more information for the health care professional. Age-appropriate distraction and diversion strategies should be used where possible. Use parents/carers where possible and appropriate; do not remove the child from parents unless necessary.

Inspection

This technique includes careful observation of the child and the skills of inspection and observation often provide the most significant data. These skills can be undertaken during the history-taking process. Always compare symmetry and adequate exposure is required.

Palpation

This technique helps to confirm inspection findings and uses the sense of touch to elicit information. Ensure your hands are warm and use a calm and gentle approach.

Percussion

The percussion technique is one whereby the skin is tapped, setting the underlying tissue in motion. The health care practitioner can then determine the density of the underlying tissue, e.g. whether the lung tissue is filled with fluid, air or solid matter (Bickley 2003). The sounds produced are called notes. The location and size of organs can also be determined, as the density of the tissue changes at the organ's borders. It is a difficult technique to master and is not always helpful in examining young children and infants.

Percussion technique (advanced technique) usually involves:

o placing the most distal joint (interphalangeal joint) of the hyper-extended middle finger of the left hand (pleximeter finger) on the body, avoiding bony tissue;
o striking this joint with the flexed middle finger of the right hand with a short, sharp strike, and often two strikes;
o removing the fingers as quickly as possible so that the sound that is generated is not dampened (Bickley 2003).

Auscultation

This technique is used to listen to the sounds of the body. The stethoscope should be:

• of the correct size, i.e. neonatal, paediatric or adult (late adolescents) to achieve skin contact and localise sounds, accessing small areas at a time;
• warm: this may be accomplished by rubbing the diaphragm and bell with a hand or bed clothing;
• clean: clean with alcohol between use.

The bell is used for low-pitched sounds:

• heart sounds: S3, S4;
• when using the bell, do not press hard as the membrane may then come in contact with the skin, thereby producing a diaphragm-like technique.

The diaphragm is used for high-pitched sounds:

- breath sounds;
- heart sounds: S1, S2, ejection click, opening snap, friction rubs;
- bowel sounds.

APPROACHES
When examining an infant:

- position the baby on the parent's lap or at least in close proximity to the parent;
- have the baby fed an hour or so prior to the examination;
- keep the environment warm;
- use a soft 'baby' tone of voice;
- smile at the baby and play;
- use a pacifier (with parental consent).

When examining a toddler:

- position the child on the parent's lap;
- ask and then instruct the parent to help with positioning for more disturbing procedures;
- promote the presence of a favourite toy/item;
- do not give a choice to the child where there is no choice; however, do give plenty of choice where there is a choice, e.g. you need to listen to the child's chest and the child's choice might consist of whether this is undertaken on the parent's lap or on the bed, before or after you listen to teddy's chest.

When examining the pre-schooler:

- the child may prefer a parent's lap or the examination table;
- pre-schoolers are usually co-operative but may not like invasive procedures;
- allow them to play with and examine any equipment you are using;
- they require short and simple explanations;
- do not give a choice to the child where there is no choice; however, do give plenty of choice where there is a choice, e.g. you need to listen to the child's chest and the child's choice

might consist of whether it is undertaken on the parent's lap or on the bed, before or after you listen to teddy's chest;

- use games to undertake examination where possible, e.g. blowing up a balloon when listening to the chest;
- tell them how well they are doing during the examination.

When examining the school-age child:

- it is usually undertaken on the examination table;
- be mindful of their increasing modesty;
- start with getting to know the child, e.g. ask about school and their friends;
- let the child examine any equipment;
- allow the child to hear or feel your findings, e.g. listen to heart beat.

When examining a young person:

- they usually do not want a parent present;
- take care not to treat as a child but also not as an adult;
- body image is important.

DOCUMENTATION

It is important to write up findings so that it is clear what you have assessed (NMC 2002) as well as to use language that is understood by the multi-disciplinary team. Notes must adhere to local policy and legal requirements:

- Write in black or blue pen.
- Write comprehensively yet succinctly, stating facts and findings.
- Record date and time.
- Provide signature and printed name of the health care professional along with designation.
- Avoid unapproved abbreviations.

SUMMARY

History-taking, physical examination and monitoring provide a comprehensive tool to assist the health care practitioner in clinical decision-making when caring for sick children and their families. Comprehensive history-taking provides a significant amount of subjective data and this is then objectively defined through the examination techniques of inspection, palpation, percussion and auscultation. Advanced communication skills and knowledge of child growth and development are essential. Accurate documentation provides the multi-disciplinary team with information on the extent of the assessment. It is commonly considered that if it is not written, it has not been done.

REFERENCES

Archer, N. & Birch, M. (1998) *Paediatric Cardiology*. Chapman and Hall Medical, London.

Bickley, L.S. (2003) *Bates Guide to Physical Examination and History Taking*, 8th edn. Lippincott, Williams and Wilkins, Philadelphia, Chapters 1 and 17.

Engel, J. (1997) *Pediatric Assessment*, 3rd edn. Mosby, St. Louis.

Farrell, P. & Sittlington, N. (2003) The baby at birth. In: Fraser, D.M. & Cooper, M.A. (eds) *Myles Textbook for Midwives*, 14th edn. Churchill Livingston, Edinburgh.

Gill, D. & O'Brien, N. (2002) *Paediatric Clinical Examination Made Easy*, 4th edn. Churchill Livingston, Edinburgh.

Goldbloom, R.B. (1997) Family interviewing and history taking. In: Goldbloom, R.B. (ed) *Pediatric Clinical Skills*, 2nd edn. Churchill Livingston, Philadelphia.

Jarvis, C. (2003) *Physical Examination and Health Assessment*. Elsevier, St. Louis, Chapter 6.

Nursing and Midwifery Council (NMC) (2002) *Guidelines for Records and Record Keeping*. NMC, London.

Wong, D. (1995) *Whaley and Wong's Nursing Care of Infants and Children*, 5th edn. Mosby, St Louis.

Respiratory Assessment 2

INTRODUCTION

Respiratory assessment in infants and children is critical in evaluating severity of illness. The history and physical assessment techniques of inspection, palpation, percussion and auscultation can be used to determine efficacy of breathing, work of breathing and adequacy of ventilation. Respiratory distress occurs primarily when there is a respiratory problem (there are other secondary causes) and the child is using all compensatory techniques available to maintain adequate ventilation and oxygenation. Once these techniques become ineffective at maintaining adequate ventilation and oxygenation (i.e. blood oxygen levels fall and blood carbon dioxide levels increase), respiratory failure occurs. Respiratory failure is the most common pathway to cardiorespiratory arrest from which there is a poor outcome (Resuscitation Council (UK) 2004). The aim of this chapter is to understand the principles of respiratory assessment for different age groups.

LEARNING OBJECTIVES

By the end of this chapter the reader will be able to:

❏ Appreciate the importance of taking a history.
❏ Outline the steps of a comprehensive assessment.
❏ Recognise symptoms of respiratory distress and respiratory failure.

HISTORY

There is often an overlap with head and neck review (see Chapter 11). The specific respiratory symptoms to ask about include:

- any previous respiratory illnesses, e.g. bronchiolitis or croup;
- any previous respiratory tests and investigations (including results), e.g. chest X-ray;
- sore throat or any difficulty swallowing;
- rhinorrhoea;
- cough: including when it occurs most, whether it is productive and if so a description of the content;
- haemoptysis: may indicate cystic fibrosis, foreign body aspiration, respiratory infection;
- fever (how often) or night sweats;
- difficulty in breathing including wheeze, croup, stridor, grunting, snoring;
- 'shortness of breath': may indicate obstruction, pulmonary oedema, pneumothorax or asthma.

(Hughes 1997)

PHYSICAL ASSESSMENT

Physical examination of the respiratory system should where possible include examination of both the anterior and posterior chest (Bickley 2003). Most of the information required in the respiratory system is gathered by effective inspection skills, particularly in the young child and infant (Gill & O'Brien 2002). Whilst maintaining adequate dignity and privacy, the child's chest needs to be naked for effective examination. It may be appropriate to ask teenage girls to displace their breasts for examination if necessary.

Inspection
(All basic skills)

Position
Observe and support the child's position of comfort. A wide variety of positions can be adopted to promote ventilation and decrease the work of breathing, e.g.

- epiglottitis – sitting upright, slightly forward and with neck extended;

- cystic fibrosis – sitting forward with arms supported on an overbed table.

Facial expression
Note the child's facial expression. When there is inadequate gas exchange even young infants can look:

- tense
- tired
- anxious (Gill & O'Brien 2002)

The child's ability to speak normally can also indicate level of 'shortness of breath', tiredness and consciousness; assess response to questions and note if the child is using stilted sentences.

Level of consciousness (see Chapter 7)
The child's level of consciousness may provide further information on:

- hypoxia – demonstrated by anxiety, restlessness, irritability;
- hypercapnoea – demonstrated by drowsiness, obtundation (Curley & Thompson 2001)

Colour
Evaluate the colour of the skin, which should be consistent with the child's ethnic background. The mucous membranes of the mouth are assessed for central colour (indicating a respiratory aetiology), whilst the nail beds of fingers and toes are observed for peripheral colour (indicating a cardiovascular aetiology). The normal colour is pink. Note that:

- cyanosis is a late sign of respiratory failure;
- mottling of the skin over the trunk and extremities often indicates inadequate tissue oxygenation;
- newborn babies may have a normal peripheral cyanosis as they adapt to extra-uterine life.

Respiratory rate and rhythm
Infants may normally have a slightly irregular breathing pattern and/or short periods of apnoea (less than 15 seconds) and

Table 2.1 Range of normal respiratory rates for different ages.

Age	Respiratory rates (per minute)
Newborn	30–60
Infant	30–60
Toddler	24–40
Child	18–30
Older child (>12 years)	12–16

Table 2.2 Definitions of abnormal respiratory patterns.

Abnormal respiratory pattern	Definition
Tachypnoea	Respiratory rate too fast
Bradypnoea	Respiratory rate too slow
Apnoea	Absent breathing
Dyspnoea	Difficult or laboured breathing
Hyperpnoea	Deep and rapid breathing
Ataxic	Unpredictable and irregular breathing

therefore respirations need to be counted for a full minute in this age group. However, apnoeas lasting longer than 15 seconds accompanied by other signs of respiratory distress are significant. Table 2.1 shows the normal range of respiratory rates (Curley & Moloney-Harmon 2001).

Tachypnoea is usually the first sign of respiratory distress (Kerem 1996), and as the child tires, the respiratory rate will decrease. Therefore a 'normalising' respiratory rate may be an ominous sign of respiratory failure. Table 2.2 outlines the definitions of abnormal respiratory patterns.

The ratio of inspiration to expiration time (I:E) ratio is normally 1:2. However:

- prolonged inspiration occurs with upper airway obstruction, e.g. croup;
- prolonged expiration occurs with lower airway obstruction, e.g. asthma.

Table 2.3 Physiology of abnormal respiratory sounds.

Abnormal respiratory sounds	Inspiratory/ expiratory	Physiology
Stridor Suggestive of upper airways disease, e.g. croup	Inspiratory	High-pitched noise due to air forced through a narrowed upper tracheal airway
Grunting Suggestive of diseases causing alveolar collapse, e.g. pneumonia (Gill & O'Brien 2002) or atelectasis *Grunting is an ominous sign*	Expiratory	Infants and young children breathe out against a partially closed glottis, attempting to increase end-expiratory pressure in the alveoli, and thereby keeping them open longer. This attempt is similar to the older child who breathes with pursed lips
Wheezing Suggestive of lower airway narrowing, e.g. asthma (SIGN/BTS 2003)	Expiratory (inspiratory and bi-phasic may also be heard)	Air is being forced out through narrowed lower airways

Respiratory sounds

The child's breathing should be quiet and effortless. When noises occur, note their characteristics and where they occur in the respiratory cycle. Table 2.3 outlines the physiology of abnormal respiratory sounds.

Chest wall shape

Infants have round chests because of the horizontal position of ribs and this imposes limitations on expansion. By school age, the chest cage resembles that of an adult. Other deformities can also limit adequate ventilation and gas exchange (Hughes 1997; Bickley 2003). Table 2.4 shows the definitions of chest deformities.

Chest expansion

Early in infancy, diaphragmatic breathing is usually observed. This means that the abdomen rises with inspiration and chest

Table 2.4 Chest deformities.

Chest deformity	Definition
Scoliosis	Lateral curvature of spine
Kyphosis	Exaggeration of normal posterior convexity of thoracic spine
Pectus carinatum	Also known as pigeon chest Sternum is more anterior Indicates chronic lung disease, e.g. asthma (SIGN/BTS 2003) or cystic fibrosis
Pectus excavatum	Also known as funnel chest Sternum is depressed
Harrison's sulcus	Depressions just below the subcostal margins Due to diaphragmatic contractions Associated with chronic airways disease
Hyperinflation	Chest becomes more barrel shaped Associated with gas trapping in the airways, e.g. bronchiolitis

expansion is minimal and then vice versa on expiration. This paradoxical breathing becomes exaggerated if the lungs become less compliant. This is often known as 'seesaw' breathing. In infancy, if there is only thoracic breathing, diaphragmatic function may be impaired.

Normal diaphragmatic breathing slowly reverses and by about 7 years of age the abdomen and chest should move together (Engel 1997). At this age if abdominal breathing becomes predominant, lung disease may be indicated.

Observe that chest expansion is equal and symmetrical and note that unequal symmetry can be associated with:

- pneumothorax
- pneumonia
- chest trauma
- atelectasis
- inhaled foreign body

Accessory muscles

When gas exchange is inadequate due to increased airway resistance (increased pressure in the airways, e.g. obstruction) or decreased lung compliance (decreased ability of the lung to expand, e.g. pneumonia), accessory muscles are used to increase the work of breathing to improve the gas exchange.

Note any of the following muscle use:

- internal and external intercostal muscles contract;
- abdominal muscles contract, causing 'abdominal breathing';
- scalene and sternocleidomastoid muscles in the neck contract to produce 'head bobbing' in infants;
- scalene and sternomastoid muscles in the neck contract in children (Hughes 1997);
- enlarging the nostrils on inspiration helps reduce airways resistance and maintains airway patency, and is known as 'nasal flaring';
- pursing of the lips in expiration maintains end-expiratory pressure within the alveoli (keeping them open) – occurs in the older child.

Chest recession

Also known as retractions, chest recession occurs in both infants and children (Curley & Thompson 2001) as a result of the increased work of breathing. The infant's soft and compliant rib cage collapses inward on inspiration with diaphragmatic contraction and then moves outward on expiration with diaphragmatic relaxation.

Upper airways disease is often associated with upper chest recession and lower airways disease with lower chest recession (Curley & Thompson 2001). Ventilation can become ineffective and therefore chest recessions are a significant sign of respiratory distress. Figure 2.1 shows where recessions can be found.

Clubbing of the finger and toe nails

Clubbing is caused by a proliferation of nail bed tissue that raises the nail's base towards the skin (Engel 1997). The finger end becomes rounded and the nail fold becomes spongy. It is associated with chronic hypoxia from either a respiratory cause or cardiac condition. The severity of clubbing is measured by the degree to which the nail bed is lifted up by the proliferation (Bickley 2003). Observe:

- the nail–skin junction and assess the angle from the lateral aspect of the digit, as shown in Fig. 2.2a (clubbing evident);
- for a diamond-shaped gap formed when the older child/young person lays the distal phalangeal joints of opposite fingers together, as shown in Fig. 2.2b (no clubbing evident).

Cough

The characteristics of a cough are important (Hughes 1997). Note the following:

- sudden or gradual onset;
- productive or non-productive;
- progressive or stagnant;
- sputum examination for colour, consistency, odour and amount. Note that infants and young children usually swallow their secretions (Gill & O'Brien 2002).

Coughing is often associated with other abnormalities, as shown in Table 2.5.

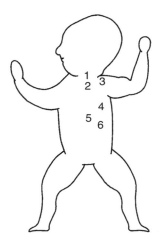

Fig. 2.1 Sites of chest recessions. 1 Tracheal tug (infant and child); 2 suprasternal (infant and child); 3 clavicular (infant and child); 4 intercostal (infant and child); 5 substernal (infant); 6 subcostal (infant and child).

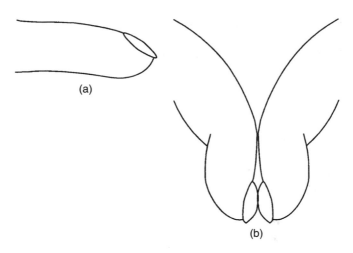

Fig. 2.2 Clubbing of the fingers. (a) Clubbing evident; (b) no clubbing evident.

Table 2.5 Cough associations.

Cough description	Indication	Sputum may be
Barking with stridor and hoarseness	Croup	
Laryngeal with hoarseness	Viral	
Dry, prolonged	Asthma	Absent, minimal
Dry, becoming rattling	Bronchitis	Large amount, smelly
Deep, unproductive	Lobar pneumonia	Absent, minimal
Deep, chesty, productive	Bronchopneumonia	Discoloured, purulent
Spasmodic, repetitive, with sudden 'whoop' on inspiration, followed by vomiting	Pertussis	Large amounts, thick, tenacious
Worse at night	May be due to a change in temperature and/or humidity	

Palpation

In infants and young children, some aspects of palpation (using hands to feel) may not be easily performed or interpreted and therefore examination must be considered within the context of the whole physical examination. Ensure that hands are warm and nails are short.

Position of trachea

(Advanced skill)

Using one finger in young children and two in older children, check that the trachea is in the midline. Deviation is not common in infants and toddlers due to mobility of trachea (Gill & O'Brien 2002). See Table 2.6 for indications of a tracheal shift.

Chest expansion

(Basic skill)

This is usually assessed adequately visually, especially in the infant and young child. However, placing hands circumferentially along the lower costal margins and assessing inspiratory expansion for adequacy and symmetry may provide further information. Ask the co-operative child to take a deep breath.

Tenderness and observed abnormalities

(Advanced skill)

Palpate over the chest and note any areas of tenderness. Assess any observed findings of lesions, bruises, scars or masses. When air enters the subcutaneous tissue, crackling, known as subcutaneous emphysema, is palpated (Hughes 1997). Causes include:

- tracheostomy formation;
- chest wound or drainage;
- severe pulmonary air-leaks, e.g. pneumomediastinum or pneumothorax.

Rhonchi or secretions may be palpated over the chest as the chest wall in younger children and infants is thin. Note any grating sensations that may indicate a pleural friction rub as the pleural layers become inflamed and rub against each other with respiration (Bickley 2003).

Table 2.6 Tracheal deviation.

Tracheal shift to the left	Tracheal shift to the right
Atelectasis on left side	Atelectasis on right side
Large pleural effusion on right side	Large pleural effusion on left side
Large pneumothorax on right side	Large pneumothorax on left side

Tactile or vocal fremitus
(Advanced skill)
You can feel the vibrations (fremitus) transmitted from the bronchopulmonary tree to the chest wall when the child speaks (ask them to say '99') or cries. To feel these vibrations:

- Place either the palms or the ulnar surface of your hands on the child's chest:
  - each side of the sternum for anterior chest examination;
  - each side of the vertebral column for posterior chest examination.
- Move symmetrically down the chest wall and then laterally to the mid-axilla line.
- Fremitus (vibrations) should be felt symmetrically (Bickley 2003).

Table 2.7 outlines increased and decreased fremitus.

Percussion
(Advanced skill)
In infants and young children, percussion may not be easily performed or interpreted and therefore examination must be

Table 2.7 Abnormal fremitus.

Increased vibrations	Decreased or absent vibrations
Over areas of consolidation, e.g. pneumonia or atelectasis	Over areas of decreased air flow, e.g. asthma, pneumothorax, pleural effusion or foreign body

considered within the context of the whole physical examination. Percussion determines whether the lung tissue is filled with fluid, air or solid matter (Bickley 2003). See Chapter 1 for the technique of percussion. Always compare sides by moving systematically from one side to the other, then to the mid-axilla region, to evaluate all lobes.

Table 2.8 shows the different percussion notes, their characteristics, where they are found normally in the body and pathological examples. Only light percussion is needed (Gill & O'Brien 2002). The sound or percussion note produced from the vibrations is usually resonant in the lungs (Bickley 2003). However, the infant's round chest normally produces a hyper-resonant pitch and resonance is reached by age 6. Therefore in the child less than 6 years of age lung resonance may indicate consolidation, e.g. atelectasis, pneumonia or pleural effusion.

Auscultation
(Basic skill)
In infants and young children, findings from auscultation may not be easily interpreted and therefore must be considered within the context of the whole physical examination.

Stethoscope
Use the diaphragm to:

- listen over the main bronchus for bronchial sounds;
- listen for the higher pitched normal bronchovesicular (in infancy) and vesicular (toddlers and children) sounds over the chest;
- auscultate the anterior and posterior chest;
- auscultate symmetrically (allows the child to act as his/her own control) and systematically over each lobe from apex to base (Hughes 1997). Figure 2.3 indicates auscultation sites in infants and children.

Breath sounds
Breath sounds are:

- usually louder in infants and young children because the thinner chest wall brings the stethoscope closer to the origin of the sounds (Engel 1997);

Table 2.8 Percussion notes.

Lung tissue	Percussion note	Intensity	Pitch	Duration	Quality	Normal example	Pathologic example
Fluid-filled	Flatness	Soft	High	Short	Flat	Thigh	Pleural effusion
Solid	Dullness	Soft to moderate	High	Moderate	Thud-like	Liver	Lung consolidation
Normal air-filled	*Resonant*	*Moderate to loud*	*Low*	*Long*	*Hollow*	*Lung fields*	*Normal*
Hyper-inflated	Hyper-resonant	Very loud	Very low	Long	Booming	—	Pneumothorax
Air-filled	Tympany	Loud	High	Moderate	Drum-like	Gastric bubble or puffed out cheek	Large pneumothorax

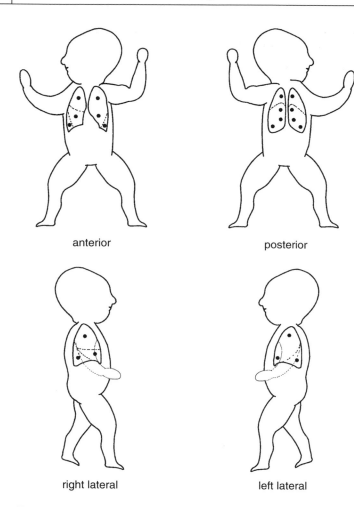

anterior

posterior

right lateral

left lateral

Fig. 2.3 Auscultation sites.

- easier to hear when the child takes bigger breaths than normal. This may be accomplished by engaging the child in games, e.g. pretending to blow out candles or blow up balloons, blow bubbles or asking the child to blow a tissue, a cotton wool ball or pinwheel.

Listen:

- between cries and try to ignore surface noises and transmitted sounds and movement;
- throughout the entire inspiratory and expiratory cycle; lifting the stethoscope too soon may result in important findings being missed;
- for normal characteristics of breath sounds (Bickley 2003), as outlined in Table 2.9;
- for normal breath sounds in normal locations, normal breath sounds in abnormal locations and the presence of added sounds.

Assess whether the breath sounds are symmetrical, normal, increased or decreased and note that:

- decreased breath sounds do occur in older children with obstructed bronchi, hyperinflated lungs, pneumothorax or pleural effusion;
- bronchial breath sounds are heard over an area of consolidation or atelectasis (demonstrating improved transmission of sound through solid or airless tissue);

Table 2.9 Normal breath sounds.

Breath sound	Characteristics
Tracheal	High pitched, loud, tubular, equal inspiratory/expiratory time over the trachea in the neck
Vesicular	Lower pitched, soft, longer inspiratory time over most of the lung field
Bronchovesicular	Intermediate pitched, intermediate sound, equal inspiratory and expiratory time in mid airway and peripheral lung fields
Bronchial	High pitched, loud, longer expiratory time over the large airways

- a child's vocalisation can often be clearly heard when the stethoscope is placed over an area of consolidation or atelectasis (Hughes 1997).

Referred breath sounds

Breath sounds are easily transmitted or 'referred' throughout the small thoracic cavity of infants and toddlers, hence the difficulty in interpretation. To assess the origin of the breath sounds originating from the upper airways as a result of secretions, place the diaphragm near the child's mouth, as referred sounds are loudest nearer their origin (Hughes 1997).

Even with a significant pneumothorax, breath sounds may be able to be heard over collapsed areas and a clear chest may have a pneumonia on chest X-ray (Gill & O'Brien 2002).

Added (or adventitious) breath sounds

Once breath sounds have been evaluated, listen for added sounds (Hughes 1997). Table 2.10 shows the characteristics of

Table 2.10 Characteristics of added breath sounds.

Added sounds	Characteristics
Crackles/crepitations (also known as rales) May be due to pneumonia, pulmonary oedema, bronchitis	Short crackling sounds on inspiration or expiration Fine crackles (fine, high-pitched, short duration) may be due to reopening of a small airway Coarse crackles (loud, bubbling, low-pitched, longer duration) may be due to air coursing through mucus, pus or fluid in large airways
Wheezes May be due to asthma	Continuous and musical on inspiration but more commonly on expiration Produced by air moving through a narrowed or obstructed airway caused by oedema, mucus or bronchospasm
Rhonchi May be related to secretions in larger airways	Low-pitched, snoring quality
Friction rub Indicates pleural rub	Harsh, grating sound with respiration Not common in pre-schoolers

added breath sounds. It is important to consider the location and timing within the respiratory cycle.

Note that wheezing occurs more commonly in infants because of the small size of their airways. Disappearance of wheeze in an asthmatic child may mean he/she is no longer moving air through narrowed airways – an ominous sign.

SUMMARY

Physical examination of the respiratory system to determine efficacy of breathing, work of breathing and adequacy of ventilation for each age group can be summarised as outlined in Tables 2.11a–c.

Table 2.11a Infant respiratory examination.

Infant	Assessment	Techniques
Efficacy of breathing	Air entry	Inspection: symmetrical chest expansion, respiratory rate Palpation: chest abnormalities Auscultation: adequate and equal inspiratory and expiratory breath sounds
	Chest movement	Inspection: symmetry, expansion, depth of inspiration
Work of breathing	Rate	Inspection
	Rhythm	Inspection
	Breath sounds/added sounds	Inspection and auscultation
	Accessory muscle use	Inspection: seesaw breathing, head bobbing, internal and external intercostal muscles, nasal flaring
	Chest recession	Inspection: tracheal tug, suprasternal, clavicular, intercostal and subcostal recession
Adequacy of ventilation	Tissue oxygenation • skin colour • mental status • cardiac assessment (heart rate)	Inspection/neurological examination: facial expression, level of consciousness Cardiovascular examination: palpation of pulses, capillary refill time, warmth of extremities

Table 2.11b Young child respiratory examination.

Young child <6 years	Assessment	Techniques
Efficacy of breathing	Air entry	Inspection: symmetrical chest expansion, respiratory rate Palpation: tenderness, tracheal position, chest abnormalities Auscultation: adequate and equal inspiratory and expiratory breath sounds
	Chest movement	Inspection: symmetry, expansion, depth of inspiration, inspiratory/expiratory ratio Palpation: symmetry, expansion
Work of breathing	Rate	Inspection
	Rhythm	Inspection
	Breath sounds/ added sounds	Inspection and auscultation
	Accessory muscle use	Inspection: internal and external intercostals, scalene and sternomastoid muscles, nasal flaring
	Chest recession	Inspection: tracheal tug, suprasternal, clavicular, and intercostals recession
Adequacy of ventilation	Tissue oxygenation • skin colour • mental status • cardiac assessment (heart rate, etc.)	Inspection/neurological examination: facial expression, level of consciousness, ability to speak Cardiovascular examination: palpation of pulses, capillary refill time, warmth of extremities
	Chest shape	Inspection
	Clubbing	Inspection

Tables 2.12a–c show normal physical examination findings, as well as some case studies showing pathological findings for different age groups.

ASSESSMENT OF AIRWAY/OXYGEN ADJUNCTS

Children and infants may require airway/oxygen adjuncts to support their oxygenation and/or ventilation (Resuscitation

Table 2.11c Older child respiratory examination.

Older child >6 years	Assessment	Techniques
Efficacy of breathing	Air entry	Inspection: symmetrical chest expansion, respiratory rate Palpation: tenderness, chest abnormalities, tracheal position, fremitus (advanced skill) Auscultation: adequate and equal inspiratory and expiratory breath sounds
	Chest movement	Inspection: symmetry, expansion, depth of inspiration, inspiratory/expiratory ratio Palpation: symmetry, expansion
Work of breathing	Rate	Inspection
	Rhythm	Inspection
	Breath sounds/ added sounds	Inspection and auscultation
	Accessory muscle use	Inspection: internal and external intercostals, scalenes and sternomastoid muscles, pursed lips
	Chest recession	Inspection: tracheal tug, suprasternal, clavicular, and intercostal recession
Adequacy of ventilation	Tissue oxygenation • skin colour • mental status • cardiac assessment (heart rate, etc.)	Inspection/neurological examination: facial expression, level of consciousness, ability to speak Cardiovascular examination: palpation of pulses, capillary refill time, warmth of extremities
	Chest shape	Inspection
	Clubbing	Inspection
	Lung density	Percussion (advanced skill): percussion notes

Council (UK) 2004). Using adjuncts effectively whilst maintaining safe application needs continuous assessment (Chandler 2001; AARC 2002).

Simple oxygen mask
Commonly used, the fractional concentration of inspired oxygen (FiO_2) varies with the patient's inspiratory flow, respiratory

Table 2.12a Infant: documentation of normal/pathological findings.

Normal
Pink centrally and peripherally
Respiratory rate 38 with good expansion bilaterally
No use of accessory muscles and no chest recession
Breath sounds bronchovesicular bilaterally; air entry equal; no added sounds

Bronchiolitis: 6-month-old
Slightly flushed centrally and pale/mottled peripherally
Miserable, crying, runny nose. Sitting on Mum's knee, won't feed
Moist cough
Respiratory rate 62 and irregular with symmetrical chest expansion
Bronchial breath sounds with prolonged expiratory time and crackles and wheezing
Nasal flaring, with intercostal and substernal recession

Croup (laryngotracheobronchitis): 12-month-old
Slightly pale centrally and peripherally
Sitting on Mum's lap, a little restless, no fever
Respiratory rate 32 with symmetrical chest expansion
Inspiratory stridor with slightly prolonged inspiratory time and barking cough
Breath sounds vesicular; equal
Slight tracheal tug, suprasternal recession and nasal flaring

pattern and mask fit, but concentration achieved can be 0.35–0.6 (35–60%). Table 2.13 shows assessment considerations of the simple oxygen mask.

Nasal prongs or cannulae
Commonly used, the FiO_2 varies with the patient's inspiratory flow but may be achieved at 0.25–0.4 (25–40%). Table 2.14 shows assessment considerations of nasal prongs or nasal cannulae.

Head box
This is used less often now; however, the FiO_2 can be controlled from 0.21 to close to 1.0 (21–100%). Table 2.15 shows assessment considerations of the head box.

Oxygen tent
This is not used very often and low levels of FiO_2 only can be achieved. Table 2.16 shows assessment considerations of the oxygen tent.

Table 2.12b Young child: documentation of normal/pathological findings.

Normal
Pink centrally and peripherally, no clubbing
Respiratory rate 25 with good expansion bilaterally
No use of accessory muscles and no chest recession
Breath sounds vesicular bilaterally; air entry equal; no added sounds

Pneumonia: 4-year-old
Slightly flushed centrally and pale/mottled peripherally
Lying supine on bed with head elevated, eyes closed but open when asked
Occasional deep cough with intermittent grunting, no clubbing
Respiratory rate 45 with dyspnoea ('It hurts')
Chest expansion decreased over left lower zone
Lower intercostal recession
Bronchial breath sounds, diminished over left lower zone with slight expiratory wheeze

Inhaled foreign body: 2-year-old
Pale centrally and peripherally
Sitting on Dad's knee, distressed and crying
Frequent coughing with some blood in the mouth
Respiratory rate 30 with unequal chest expansion (decreased on left side)
Suprasternal recession and nasal flaring
Vesicular breath sounds (decreased) with inspiratory wheeze

Table 2.12c Older child: documentation of normal/pathological findings.

Normal
Pink centrally and peripherally, no clubbing
Respiratory rate 20 with good expansion bilaterally
No use of accessory muscles and no chest recession
Lungs resonant (advanced skill)
Breath sounds vesicular bilaterally; air entry equal; no added sounds

Acute asthma: 10-year-old
Pale centrally and peripherally
Sitting supine against raised head of bed. Restless but sleepy, some difficulty speaking – only two- to three-word sentences, feels sick and has a tight chest
Chest wall normal shape, no clubbing
Dry, prolonged coughing episodes
Respiratory rate 28 and slightly laboured
Chest expansion decreased bilaterally
Some intercostals recession and use of sternomastoids
Prolonged expiration with loud inspiratory and expiratory wheeze
Trachea in mid-line; decreased fremitus in lower zones (advanced skill)
Slightly hyper-resonant throughout (advanced skill)

Table 2.13 Assessment of a simple oxygen mask.

Check:
- gas flow against the prescription;
- gas flow should be greater than/equal to 6 L to prevent rebreathing of expired air (holes on each side of the mask provide an exit for exhaled gases; room air may also be entrained);
- the right sized mask is used (neonatal for infants, paediatric for children, adult for young people);
- the child tolerates the mask (infants and young children tolerate it less);
- the skin around the ear and face for pressure from the elastic strap;
- the child's face and eyes for pressure from the mask;
- for the accumulation of moisture in the mask or on the face;
- for any vomiting that can cause aspiration;
- humidification of the gas (if /as per local policy).

Table 2.14 Assessment of nasal prongs or cannulae.

Check:
- gas flow against the prescription:
  - gas flow should not exceed child's own predicted minute volume
  - predicted minute volume = 7 ml/kg × respiratory rate
  - e.g. a 10-kg child breathing at 20 breaths/min will have a predicted minute volume of 1.4 L; therefore maximum gas flow should not exceed 1.4 L
  - use a local protocol
    - e.g. under 2 years of age – up to 2 L gas flow
    - over 2 years of age – up to 4 L gas flow
- the appropriate size (neonatal for infants, paediatric for children, adult for young people) inserted into the patient's nares comfortably;
- the tubing is kept away from the infant's neck to prevent airway obstruction;
- the skin around the nose for pressure;
- the child's tolerance of the device (child can become irritable with high gas flows);
- the child is not primarily breathing through the mouth and thereby losing much of the gas flow;
- the securing strategy of the tubing on the face for security, pressure, allergic reaction and skin integrity;
- the child's abdomen for distension from air entering the stomach;
- the child for vomiting from air entering the stomach;
- the child's nose for nasal secretions which may obstruct gas flow;
- adequate humidification (if used, as per local policy);
- these are not being used in children with nasal obstruction;
- the young infant's work of breathing as infants are obligatory nose breathers and obstruction to nasal passages can impede ventilation.

Table 2.15 Assessment of head box.

Check:
- oxygen percentage given against prescription;
- there is sufficient gas flow to prevent carbon dioxide buildup within the box (gas flow > 3 L/kg);
- oxygen analyser is calibrated (as per local protocol) with alarms set;
- oxygen analyser sensor is placed near to the infant's nose and mouth so that FiO_2 may be measured most accurately for the patient;
- warm and moist wet humidification is maintained to prevent drying and cooling of airways;
- if misting of the box does occur (should not with adequate humidification), carry out frequent demisting to ensure adequate observation;
- temperature inside the box to prevent overheating or heat loss of the infant;
- an appropriate sized box is used (the infant's head should fit comfortably but should not allow the infant to wriggle out of the box);
- there are no air leaks around the edges of the box except at the infant's neck;
- the infant's neck is not subject to pressure from the box.

Table 2.16 Assessment of oxygen tent.

Check:
- oxygen percentage given against prescription;
- the tent fits around the bed;
- the tent for temperature and moisture;
- the tent is not being opened too often, thereby losing the FiO_2.

Oxygen mask with reservoir bag

This is used in an emergency and with impending respiratory failure. With a snug fit, the FiO_2 should reach 0.95 (95%). Table 2.17 shows assessment considerations of the oxygen mask with reservoir bag.

The bag-valve-mask ventilation circuit (self-inflating)

This is used to provide oxygen and ventilation to the child/ infant. O_2 concentrations up to 0.95 (95%) can be achieved with the oxygen reservoir attached. Without the oxygen reservoir, it drops to 0.50 (50%).

This circuit must not be used to provide 'blow-by' oxygen as there is limited oxygen flow through the valve when the circuit

Table 2.17 Assessment of oxygen mask with reservoir bag.

Check:
- gas flow against the prescription;
- gas flow should be at the level to maintain the reservoir full (usually 10–15 L);
  - ○ one-way valves ensure fresh oxygen is continually supplied with no mixing of expired gases in the reservoir
  - ○ there is minimal room air entrainment
- the child tolerates the mask;
- the skin around the ear and face for pressure from the elastic;
- the child's face and eyes for pressure from the mask;
- should be first-line use in resuscitation procedures.

Table 2.18 Assessment of bag-valve-mask ventilation circuit (self-inflating).

Check:
- the circuit is correctly assembled, including the oxygen reservoir;
- has an oxygen outlet available/attached (as per local protocol);
- has a mask appropriate to the size of the child
  - ○ from bridge of nose to cleft of chin
- the correct size bag is used (250 ml for infants, 450–500 ml for children, 1600–2000 ml for older children/young people).

is not being manually inflated (Carter *et al.* 2005). Table 2.18 shows assessment considerations of the bag-valve-mask ventilation circuit.

Anaesthetic/flow-inflating circuits
These are found mainly in critical care areas and can provide the operator with information about the child's/infant's lung compliance. Table 2.19 shows assessment considerations of the anaesthetic/flow-inflating circuit.

The oro-pharyngeal airway
This is used to maintain the airway of the child with a decreased level of consciousness. Table 2.20 shows assessment considerations of the oro-pharyngeal airway.

Table 2.19 Assessment of anaesthetic/flow-inflating circuits.

Check:
- the circuit is correctly assembled;
- there is an oxygen outlet available;
- oxygen flows through the circuit but must flow at more than three times the child's minute ventilation (>30 ml/kg) to prevent rebreathing;
- the open-end of the 500-ml circuit is able to be manipulated and the bag fills when occluded;
- the 1-L and 2-L bags may have a valve to control gas flow;
- there is a mask appropriate to the size of the child
  ○ from bridge of nose to cleft of chin
- the correct size bag is used (500 ml for infants and young children, 1 L for older children and 2 L for young people).

Table 2.20 Assessment of the oro-pharyngeal airway.

Check:
- the child is not vomiting (may cause aspiration);
- the child does not have any signs of laryngospasm
  ○ stridor
  ○ closing airway (no lung gas flow)
- there is minimal pressure to the lips, tongue, teeth and soft tissue.

Remove when the child's conscious level improves or when the child attempts to spit the airway out.

An oro-pharyngeal airway may be used in the child who is biting on his/her endotracheal tube. This should be a short-term measure and a bite-block may be more appropriate.

The oro-pharyngeal tube is sized by holding the tube near to the child's mouth with one end at the angle of the jaw and ensuring that the other end is at the centre of the incisors (or where they will be).

The naso-pharyngeal airway

This may be used in the child requiring airway maintenance but who might be regaining consciousness. Table 2.21 shows assessment considerations of the naso-pharyngeal airway.

The tracheostomy tube

Tracheostomies are usually used for long-term airway maintenance. Table 2.22 shows assessment considerations of the tracheostomy tube.

Table 2.21 Assessment of the naso-pharyngeal airway.

Check the child for:
- blanching of the nares;
- ulceration of the nares;
- the safety pin, if used (used particularly when a shortened endotracheal tube is used in small children and infants), is fastened and not in contact with the skin;
- epistaxis;
- laryngospasm
  ○ stridor
  ○ closing airway

Table 2.22 Assessment of the tracheostomy tube (Tamburri 2000; Wilson 2005).

Check:
- replacement tubes are easily available, including one size smaller tube and one size larger, usually at the bedside;
- emergency equipment is readily available (as per local protocol), usually including tracheal dilators, endotracheal intubation equipment, oxygen and suction capabilities, tapes, scissors;
- the cuff pressure/volume is maintained (as per local protocol) by checking volume with a syringe or pressure with a pressure monitor;
- the wound site is clean, not bleeding, and with no signs of infection;
- a dressing is used if the tracheostomy site is oozing or being rubbed;
- the surrounding skin is not exposed to pressure or rubbing from the tube;
- the tapes are secure; firm but not tight (can fit two fingers between the tape and skin); they are dry and not rubbing. Inspect all of neck including skin folds in infants;
- the skin in and around the tracheostomy site is not becoming granulated; seek medical opinion in management.

The endotracheal tube (ETT)

Intubating children provides a secure airway for controlling ventilation and oxygenation. Table 2.23 shows assessment considerations of the ETT.

The ventilator

The ventilator is a machine that is able to artificially provide ventilation and oxygenation for the patient either partially or

Table 2.23 Assessment of the endotracheal tube (ETT).

Check that the following is immediately available:
- oxygen delivery system including hand ventilation circuit;
- suction system including appropriately sized suction and yankeur suckers:
  - ○ catheter sizes may be calculated by
    - – doubling the size of the ETT, e.g. ETT size 4 = size 8 Fg catheter
    - – referring to a published/local chart
- replacement tubes, including one size larger and one size smaller:
  - ○ tube size may be estimated by
    - – premature infants: 2.5–3.0 mm
    - – term infants: 3.0–3.5 mm
    - – infants under 1 year: 4.0–4.5 mm
    - – children over 1 year: calculating age of patient (in years) ÷ 4 + 4
    - – the diameter of the child's little finger roughly reflects the size of the tube required (not reliable)
- endotracheal intubation equipment and drug therapy (e.g. benzodiazepines, chemical paralysis, narcotic analgesia);
- monitoring equipment (minimal pulse oximetry and heart rate, usually also ECG, blood pressure and often $ETCO_2$).

Check the ETT:
- cuff pressure/volume is maintained (as per local protocol) by checking volume with a syringe or pressure with a pressure monitor (when used);
- maintains alignment and is not kinked;
- is secured effectively;
- is not able to move/minimal movement within the airway;
- for air leak from around the tube (audible on ventilatory inspiration or when manually ventilated);
- is not being pulled by the weight of the ventilator tubing; secure/support tubing with a ventilator arm or weight;
- for displacement (is there adequate chest expansion); remove if ETT has dislodged
- for obstruction (is there adequate chest expansion); perform airway clearance with manual ventilation and suctioning as indicated.

Check the child:
- that his/her head is in neutral position (as far as possible);
- that his/her mouth and nose are not exposed to pressure and ulceration;
- that skin is intact (no allergic reactions) around the security strapping (protective dressing, e.g. duoderm may have been used);
- is not able to self-extubate (use appropriate restraint, e.g. adequate sedation).

Table 2.24 Assessment of the ventilator.

Check:
- the settings correlate with the prescription;
- alarm settings are appropriate; you need to decide at what point do I want to be alerted to a change in parameter, and set alarms accordingly;
- humidification temperature and water level are correct (if used);
- heat and moisture exchange (HME) device is changed (if used) as per local protocol;
- tubing is leak and water free;
- documentation includes those patient parameters that alter with change in respiratory status, e.g. in volume-controlled ventilation, pressure values should be monitored. In pressure-controlled ventilation, tidal/minute volume values should be monitored.

wholly. Table 2.24 shows assessment considerations of the ventilator.

REFERENCES

American Association of Respiratory Care (AARC) (2002) Selection of an oxygen delivery device for neonatal and pediatric patients. *Respiratory Care*, **47** (6), 707–716.

Bickley, L.S. (2003) *Bates Guide to Physical Examination and History Taking*, 8th edn. Lippincott, Williams and Wilkins, Philadelphia, Chapters 6 and 17.

Carter, B.G., Fairbank, B., Tibbals, J., Hochman, M. & Osborne, A. (2005) Oxygen delivery using self-inflating resuscitation bags. *Pediatric Critical Care Medicine*, **6** (2), 125–128.

Chandler, T. (2001) Oxygen administration. *Paediatric Nursing*, **13** (8), 37–42.

Curley, M.A.Q. & Moloney-Harmon, P.A. (2001) *Critical Care Nursing of Infants and Children*, 2nd edn. W.B. Saunders, Philadelphia, pp 233–308.

Curley, M.A.Q. & Thompson, J.E. (2001) Oxygenation and ventilation. In: Curley, M.A.Q. & Moloney-Harmon, P.A. (eds) *Critical Care Nursing of Infants and Children*, 2nd edn. W.B. Saunders, Philadelphia, pp 233–308.

Engel, J. (1997) *Pediatric Assessment*, 3rd edn. Mosby, St. Louis.

Gill, D. & O'Brien, N. (2002) *Paediatric Clinical Examination Made Easy*, 4th edn. Churchill Livingston, Edinburgh.

Hughes, A.H. (1997) Evaluating the child's respiratory system. In: Goldbloom, R.B. (ed) *Pediatric Clinical Skills*, 2nd edn. Churchill Livingston, Philadelphia, pp 171–191.

Kerem, E. (1996) Why do infants and small children breathe faster? *Pediatric Pulmonology*, **21**, 65–68.

Resuscitation Council (UK) (2004) *European Paediatric Life Support Course Provider Manual*. Resuscitation Council (UK), London.

Scottish Intercollegiate Guideline Network and British Thoracic Society (SIGN/BTS) (2003) British guideline on the management of asthma. *Thorax*, **58** (Suppl. I).

Tamburri, L.M. (2000) Care of the patient with a tracheostomy. *Orthopaedic Nursing*, **19** (2), 49–60.

Wilson, M. (2005) Paediatric tracheostomy. *Paediatric Nursing*, **17** (3), 38–44.

3 | Respiratory Monitoring

INTRODUCTION

Technology can be a useful aid to physical examination in monitoring the child's response to therapy and progress, but it does not replace these skills. Despite the readings from these adjuncts, the child must always also be physically assessed, as discussed in Chapters 1 and 2. Techniques for monitoring need to be correctly and safely used to ensure accurate readings.

LEARNING OBJECTIVES

By the end of this chapter the reader will be able to:

❑ Appreciate the range of monitoring techniques commonly available.
❑ Understand the effective and safe use of monitoring.
❑ Learn practical skills in using monitoring.

PULSE OXIMETRY

Pulse oximetry has become one of the most frequently used respiratory monitoring technological tools in recent times. It provides information about the oxygenation status of the child and infant and:

- is non-invasive;
- does not require calibration;
- does not require specific skin preparation;
- may be portable;
- can provide either spot checks or continuous monitoring;
- has been found to decrease the need for so much arterial blood gas sampling (Milner & Hull 1998).

What it measures

Pulse oximetry (SpO_2) measures the percentage of oxygen saturation of haemoglobin in arterial blood as measured by pulse oximetry (Chandler 2000). SpO_2 readings cannot be compared with the arterial blood gas (ABG) analysis (Moyle 1999) as this provides an estimate of SaO_2 (measures the percentage of oxygen saturation of haemoglobin in arterial blood as measured by co-oximetry). Below 70% the readings are less accurate (Grap 2002), but above this manufacturers generally claim accuracy within 3%.

Estimation of oxygen saturation is undertaken by two light-emitting diodes (LEDS) at 660 nm (red) and 940 nm (near infrared) that illuminate alternately at high frequencies. A photodetector on the other side of the probe measures the intensity of each wavelength being transmitted through the tissue during the cardiac cycle and so the probe needs a constant influx of arterial blood. This information is sent to the computer where an algorithm compares the ratio of the pulsatile change of the red light to the infrared light during the cardiac cycle. Oxyhaemoglobin absorbs more of the near infrared light (Grap 2002).

Although pulse oximetry has been found to be useful in detecting hypoxaemia, it does not provide information on the effectiveness of ventilation or carbon dioxide retention (Grap 2002). Children and infants with some congenital cardiac defects will have low SpO_2 as a normal value for them. Oxygen therapy and SpO_2 alarm limits will need to be administered/set appropriately. Pre-term infants are at risk of hyperoxaemia. Alarm limits will need to be set appropriately (the upper alarm limit is usually set at 95%) (Bohnhorst *et al*. 2002). Note that in infants with right to left cardiac shunting, the right hand can be used for pre-ductal SpO_2 measures and the left hand or foot for post-ductal SpO_2 measures (Curley & Thompson 2001).

Probes and probe sites
- Probe sites need to be clean, pulsatile and preferably without nail varnish.
- The probe needs to be clean and secured firmly but not tight (Smith 1995), as per manufacturer instructions.

- Using extra tape is discouraged (Moyle 1999) as it can:
  - affect accuracy as it may cause venous flow in the area to become pulsatile
  - increase the risk of pressure damage
  - increase the risk of thermal damage
- Possible probe positions include:
  - fingers (false readings when the probe is placed beyond the fingertip)
  - palms
  - feet (useful in infants) (Grap 2002)
  - toes
  - ear lobe
  - nose bridge
  - forehead
- Adult probes should not be used on a small child/infant (Moyle 1999) because:
  - the energy sources are too far apart, therefore affecting accuracy
  - there is a greater risk of thermal injury as more energy is used
  - pressure points may develop due to ill-fitting probes
  - the LEDS may not pass through vascular bed
- Change the site of the probe:
  - as per manufacturer's instructions
  - following assessment of the skin integrity
  - usually 4–6 hourly in children
  - maybe more frequently (e.g. 2 hourly) in infants due to their thinner skin.

Oxygen saturation monitors

Hand-held monitors can be used for one-off or spot checks of the patient's SpO_2; however, they do not always capture the continuous trends nor have the more extensive features on continuous monitoring machines (Chandler 2000). Check:

- alarm settings: the practitioner needs to decide at what point he/she wants to know the reading has changed, and set the alarms accordingly;

- the machine is plugged in so the battery is charging (Chandler 2000);
- for an adequate trace on the screen (Chandler 2000) – a plethysmographic waveform or bar indicating strength. How strong the patient's pulse is will determine the amplitude of the waveform (Slota 1998). Figure 3.1 shows a plethysmographic waveform and a bar graph.
- whether it is necessary to compare the pulse rate on the child with the pulse reading on the saturation monitor;
- that the LEDS are shining downwards where possible and the light source and photodetector are opposing one another (Chandler 2000);
- that the lead is secured against the skin proximally, without causing pressure to the patient;
- that the clinical condition correlates with the SpO_2 results.

Impact on the accuracy of SpO_2 readings

Table 3.1 shows some conditions and issues that will have an impact on the accuracy of SpO_2 readings.

ARTERIAL BLOOD GASES (ABG)

ABG analysis is considered to be the gold standard in determining the patient's acid–base balance (Yildizdas *et al.* 2004).

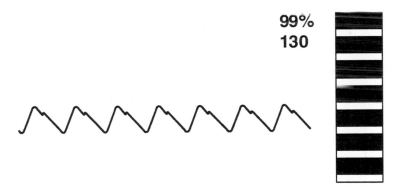

Fig. 3.1 An ideal plethysmographic waveform and a bar graph.

Table 3.1 Patient conditions and issues impacting on the accuracy of SpO_2 readings.

Phenomena	Impact
Carboxyhaemoglobin (Moyle 1999)	Over-reading Reads carboxyhaemoglobin as oxyhaemoglobin Carboxyhaemoglobin can be as a result of breathing cigarette smoke, traffic fumes or smoke inhalation
Methaemoglobin (Moyle 1999)	Under-reading Affects the calibration Methaemoglobin can be present as a result of drugs, e.g. nitric oxide
Blood disorders, e.g. thalassaemia or sickle cell disease	May alter the readings
IV dye administration, e.g. methylene blue	May give false high readings
High lipid levels	May alter the readings
Child mobility (Moyle 1999)	Causes a change in the light absorption The detector may not be able to measure these
Child has decreased perfusion of the limbs (Jevon & Ewens 2002)	Inaccurate readings as the pulse oximeter needs the pulsation of arterial blood entering the probe site. Shock or hypothermia may cause hypoperfusion Some cardiac arrhythmias, e.g. supraventricular tachycardia may cause a decrease in cardiac output and therefore perfusion
Venous pulsations (Curley & Maloney-Harmon 2001)	Inaccurate readings Can occur when sensor is placed on a dependent limb or during decreased venous return states, e.g. increased intrathoracic pressure (positive pressure ventilation) or congestive heart failure
Infant receiving phototherapy or any other strong ambient light sources (Curley & Maloney-Harmon 2001)	Photodetector cannot differentiate between sources of light May over-read Covering the probe site may help to obliterate these other sources of light
Child's limb is oedematous	May cause scattering of light before it reaches the detector Inaccurate readings
Child is anaemic	Haemoglobin must be the predominant colorant of the blood May provide false high readings
The young person has nail polish on (Cote *et al.* 1988)	Certain colours have been found to interfere with readings, e.g. black/blue/brown/red
Non-invasive blood pressure cuff on same limb as SpO_2 probe (Smith 1995)	Interferes with continuous readings during inflation and deflation

Although it provides information on oxygenation (PaO_2) and ventilation status (pH and $PaCO_2$) the results must be analysed in line with the patient's clinical condition.

Sampling

The sample of arterial blood may be drawn by means of:

- a cannula situated in an artery (frequently the radial artery but may be brachial, femoral, umbilical or axilla);
- an arterial stab (usually radial or femoral); arteries lie deeper than veins and this procedure is painful;
- a capillary prick (ear lobe or heel) – not accurate as it is mixed arterial and venous blood.

Sampling technique

See Transducers in Chapter 5.

Assessment of arterial blood gas puncture sites

Look for:

- and provide adequate analgesia (where appropriate) for artery puncturing (Sado & Deakin 2005);
- and consider evaluating ulnar arterial flow (using the 'Allen' test) prior to puncturing the radial artery to ensure arterial blood flow to the digits is not compromised, although this test is not routinely used due to poor sensitivity and specificity for radial artery puncture complications (Steele 1999);
- signs of bleeding and haematoma after compressing the site for at least 5 minutes (or longer in anticoagulated patients) after puncture (Sheehy & Lombardi 1995);
- and evaluate capillary refill time (CRT), colour and warmth of digits indicating adequate arterial blood flow prior to and following arterial puncture/cannula placement.

Managing the sample

- If it has not been drawn directly into a heparinised syringe, it should be injected into a heparinised sample pot immediately.
- It should be analysed at room temperature within 15 minutes because gas exchange and metabolism continues and may affect accuracy (Beaumont 1997).

- After 15 minutes, the sample should be cooled to reduce metabolism. Cool water is recommended rather than ice as ice may cause haemolysis and hence inaccurate results (Woodrow 2004).
- Delays in analysis may also lead to inaccurate results due to the separation of cells and plasma; the sample should therefore be rolled gently to maintain mixing but not shaken as this may cause haemolysis (Woodrow 2004).

Blood gas analysis machine

There may be a local protocol to input the patient's temperature to the blood gas analyser to compensate for the effect of temperature on the solubility of gases (Simpson 2004). However, although there are no known reference ranges for parameters when the temperature has been corrected, it is thought that measured parameters (PaO_2 and $PaCO_2$) may be lower in the pyrexial patient and higher in the hypothermic patient (Martin 1999). Temperature correction policy needs deciding within each unit so that trends (rather than absolutes) can be monitored.

(*Note what your clinical area policy is:*)

Depending on local protocol, the use of the ABG machine may also require a user code or password and patient information, e.g. patient number. Current risk management training also dictates that staff have the appropriately approved training to use the machine.

Different blood gas machines have abilities to measure and calculate different parameters (Woodrow 2004). Electrolyte (sodium, potassium, chloride, bicarbonate, glucose, ionised magnesium and calcium), metabolite (methaemoglobin, lactate) and oxygen saturation measurements (the saturation of oxygen in the arterial blood as measured by co-oximetry) can also be provided by blood gas analysis machines. For the purposes of this book, the following will be discussed:

- pH: the hygrogen ion (H^+) concentration is a *measured* parameter.
- $PaCO_2$: the partial pressure of carbon dioxide dissolved in arterial blood is a *measured* parameter.

- PaO_2: the partial pressure of oxygen dissolved in arterial blood is a *measured* parameter.
- HCO_3-: bicarbonate is *calculated* from the above parameters (RCH 2003).
- BE: indicates the level of base (alkali) in the blood and is *calculated* from the above parameters.

The main standard unit of blood gases in the UK is the kilopascal (kPa) (Simpson 2004). In other countries millimetres of mercury (mmHg) may be used. The following are conversions (Jevon & Ewens 2002):

$$1 \text{ kPa} = 7.5 \text{ mmHg}$$
$$1 \text{ mmHg} = 0.133 \text{ kPa}$$

to convert kPa to mmHg   multiply kPa by 7.5
to convert mmHg to kPa   divide mmHg by 7.5

Purposes for ABG analysis

Note that exact reference ranges for ABG parameters vary from unit to unit. The following ranges are only one set used in one clinical area.

(*The reader is invited to write in local values:*)

Assessing oxygenation

- Oxygen in a gaseous state:

     Normal PaO_2 values: (*Reader's clinical area values:*)
     Neonate: 7.2–12.6 kPa
     Child: 11.0–14.4 kPa

- Oxygen carried on Hb:

     Normal SaO_2 values: 95–100%
     Pulse oximetry has been previously discussed.

- Higher than normal PaO_2 and SaO_2 values usually indicate unnecessarily high levels of oxygen administration and it should be reduced. Oxygen toxicity is a risk for infants (retinopathy of prematurity in pre-term infants) and children (lung fibrosis).

- Lower than normal levels usually indicate hypoxaemia (low levels of oxygen in the blood).

PaO_2 and SaO_2 results must take into account the oxygen therapy at the time. If a child is just maintaining normal PaO_2 but is on high levels of oxygen therapy, it indicates an ongoing oxygenation problem.

Assessing the acid–base balance
pH
The hydrogen ion concentration measures the acidity/alkalinity of the blood and a small change in pH can dramatically alter the hydrogen ion concentration (pH expresses the negative logarithm of H^+). The blood pH needs to be maintained within limited parameters for normal cell function, and outwith a pH of 6.8–7.8, survival is unlikely.

> Normal values: (*Reader's clinical area values:*)
> Neonate: 7.29–7.45
> Child: 7.35–7.45

The blood has systems to maintain this pH (Simpson 2004):

- Buffers are weak acids or bases that are able to help control pH by taking up or releasing H^+.
- The lungs help to control pH by altering the amount of CO_2 present (CO_2 is a potential acid as it combines with water to form carbonic acid and is a major source of acid).
- The kidneys can help, but this is a slower process in compensating for abnormal pH.

Analysing the pH:

- if the pH rises above 7.45, alkalosis is present;
- if the pH falls below 7.35 (or in neonates 7.29), acidosis is present.

The first thing to look at in an ABG result is the pH:

- Is it normal (between 7.35 and 7.45)?
- Does it indicate alkalosis (above 7.45) or acidosis (below 7.35)?

Acid–base balance is affected by both respiratory and metabolic processes. To determine which is the cause of any abnormal pH, look first to the respiratory processes, i.e. the $PaCO_2$.

$PaCO_2$

Carbon dioxide is produced by body cells as a waste product of metabolism. Hypo- and hypercapnoea (low and high levels of carbon dioxide) stimulate the respiratory centre in the brainstem to slow down and increase respiratory rate and depth respectively to maintain a normal range in the blood:

> Normal values: (*Reader's clinical area values:*)
> Neonate: 3.6–5.3 kPa
> Child: 4.3–6.4 kPa

Hypoventilation

- Respiratory disease or abnormalities may lead to hypoventilation and an inability to remove the carbon dioxide.
- The $PaCO_2$ will therefore rise, causing an acidosis. The pH would fall below the normal (below 7.35).
- This acidosis would therefore be known as a *respiratory acidosis* because the low pH can be seen to have a respiratory cause.

Hyperventilation

- Is less often seen and usually as a result of over-ventilation or as a compensatory mechanism.
- In this case, the $PaCO_2$ would drop below normal limits, causing an alkalosis. The pH would rise above normal levels (above 7.45).
- This alkalosis would therefore be known as a *respiratory alkalosis* because the high pH can be seen to have a respiratory cause.

The second thing to look at in an ABG result is the $PaCO_2$:

- Is the $PaCO_2$ within normal limits (4.3–6.4)?
- If the pH is abnormal, can it be due to a respiratory cause?

HCO₃

- Bicarbonate is the main chemical buffer in the blood and so the levels indicate the metabolic acid–base status.

> Normal standard levels: (*Reader's clinical area values:*)
> 21.0–28.0 mmol/L

- High levels of HCO_3 indicate a metabolic alkalosis.
- Low levels of HCO_3 indicate a metabolic acidosis.

The third thing to look at in an ABG result is the HCO₃:

- Is the HCO_3 within normal limits?
- Does it indicate an acidosis or alkalosis?

BE

Base excess (BE) is not a requirement to determine acid–base balance. It usually follows the trends of the HCO_3 values.

> Normal values: (*Reader's clinical area values:*)
> Neonate: −10 to −2
> Child: −4 to +2
> Older child: −3 to +3

Because it indicates the level of base in the blood:

- a high level suggests metabolic alkalosis (above +3);
- a low level suggests metabolic acidosis (below −3).

The fourth thing to look at in an ABG result is the BE:

- Is the BE within normal limits (−3 to +3)?
- Does it indicate an acidosis or alkalosis?

Interpreting uncompensated acid–base balance disturbances

These have an abnormal pH and one abnormal parameter (either the $PaCO_2$ or the HCO_3) indicating the cause. Table 3.2 shows the range of uncompensated acid–base disturbances.

Compensation

In the healthy person, an imbalance of either the respiratory or metabolic function can be compensated for by the other.

Table 3.2 The range of uncompensated acid–base disturbances. (Note: an oblique mark in the table indicates the values for the neonate/child.)

pH	PaCO$_2$	HCO$_3$/BE	Imbalance/cause	ABG example
Decreased (<7.35)	Increased (>5.3/6.4)	Normal (21–28) (–3 to +3)	**Respiratory acidosis** Any causes of respiratory or neurological compromise or failure, e.g. asthma, sedation, head injury	pH 7.22 PaCO$_2$ 8.6 PaO$_2$ 10.5 HCO$_3$ 24 BE +2
Increased (>7.45)	Decreased (<3.6/4.3)	Normal (21–28) (–3 to +3)	**Respiratory alkalosis** Any causes of excess ventilation, e.g. hysterical hyperventilation, over-mechanical ventilation	pH 7.52 PaCO$_2$ 2.8 PaO$_2$ 10.5 HCO$_3$ 24 BE +2
Decreased (<7.35)	Normal (3.6–5.3/4.3–6.4)	Decreased (<21) (<–3/–10)	**Metabolic acidosis** Any causes of excess acid production or alkaline loss, e.g. sepsis, diabetic ketoacidosis, diarrhoea	pH 7.22 PaCO$_2$ 5.1 PaO$_2$ 10.5 HCO$_3$ 15 BE –10
Increased (>7.45)	Normal (3.6–5.3/4.3–6.4)	Increased (>28) (>–2/+3)	**Metabolic alkalosis** Any causes of a loss of acids or increased alkalines, e.g. severe vomiting, diuretics	pH 7.52 PaCO$_2$ 5.1 PaO$_2$ 10.5 HCO$_3$ 38 BE +12

However, although respiratory compensation is fairly quick (increase/decrease rate and depth of breathing), metabolic processes take longer (buffer systems) in their attempt to normalise the pH (Simpson 2004).

Respiratory acidosis with metabolic compensation

The HCO_3 levels will increase to try to make the blood more alkalotic in order to compensate for the acidosis. The kidneys excrete acid but retain HCO_3. This will shift the pH towards normal, providing a partial compensation. Eventually, a normal pH will be achieved, producing a full compensation. Table 3.3 shows the metabolic compensation mechanism and Table 3.4 shows a blood gas analysis example of respiratory acidosis with and without compensation.

Respiratory alkalosis with metabolic compensation

The HCO_3 levels will decrease to try to make the blood more acidotic in order to compensate for the alkalosis. The kidneys reduce reabsorption of HCO_3 and increase excretion. This will shift the pH towards normal, providing a partial compensation. Eventually, a normal pH will be achieved, producing full compensation. Table 3.5 shows the metabolic compensation

Table 3.3 The metabolic compensation mechanism.

Parameters	Partial compensation	Full compensation
pH	Decreased but will be moving towards normal	Normal
$PaCO_2$	(Already) increased	(Already) increased
HCO_3	Increased (having been normal)	Increased (having been normal)

Table 3.4 Respiratory acidosis with and without compensation.

Respiratory acidosis uncompensated	Respiratory acidosis with metabolic compensation
pH 7.22	pH 7.35
$PaCO_2$ 8.6	$PaCO_2$ 8.0
PaO_2 10.5	PaO_2 10.5
HCO_3 24	HCO_3 32
BE +2	BE +6

mechanism and Table 3.6 shows a blood gas analysis example of respiratory alkalosis with and without compensation.

Metabolic acidosis with respiratory compensation

The $PaCO_2$ will decrease to try to make the blood more alkalotic in order to compensate for the acidosis. The lungs will hyperventilate. This will shift the pH towards normal, providing a partial compensation. Eventually, a normal pH will be achieved, producing full compensation. Table 3.7 shows the respiratory compensation mechanism and Table 3.8 shows a blood gas analysis example of metabolic acidosis with and without compensation.

Metabolic alkalosis with respiratory compensation

The $PaCO_2$ will increase to try to make the blood more acidotic in order to compensate for the alkalosis. The lungs will hypoventilate. This will shift the pH towards normal, providing a partial compensation. Eventually, a normal pH will be achieved,

Table 3.5 The metabolic compensation mechanism.

Parameter	Partial compensation	Full compensation
pH	Increased but will be moving towards normal	Normal
$PaCO_2$	(Already) decreased	(Already) decreased
HCO_3	Decreased (having been normal)	Decreased (having been normal)

Table 3.6 Respiratory alkalosis with and without compensation.

Respiratory alkalosis uncompensated	Respiratory alkalosis with metabolic compensation
pH 7.52	pH 7.45
$PaCO_2$ 2.8	$PaCO_2$ 3.0
PaO_2 10.5	PaO_2 10.5
HCO_3 24	HCO_3 15
BE +2	BE −7

Table 3.7 The respiratory compensation mechanism.

Parameter	Partial compensation	Full compensation
pH	Decreased but will be moving towards normal	Normal
$PaCO_2$	Decreased (having been normal)	Decreased (having been normal)
HCO_3	(Already) decreased	(Already) decreased

Table 3.8 Metabolic acidosis with and without compensation.

Metabolic acidosis uncompensated	Metabolic acidosis with respiratory compensation
pH 7.22	pH 7.35
$PaCO_2$ 5.1	$PaCO_2$ 2.8
PaO_2 10.5	PaO_2 10.5
HCO_3 15	HCO_3 14
BE −10	BE −9

Table 3.9 The respiratory compensation mechanism.

Parameter	Partial compensation	Full compensation
pH	Increased but will be moving towards normal	Normal
$PaCO_2$	Increased (having been normal)	Increased (having been normal)
HCO_3	(Already) increased	(Already) increased

producing full compensation. Table 3.9 shows the respiratory compensation mechanism and Table 3.10 shows a blood gas analysis example of metabolic alkalosis with and without compensation.

Mixed disorders

There may be both respiratory and metabolic abnormal pathologies occurring. In full compensation where there is a normal

Table 3.10 Metabolic alkalosis with and without compensation.

Metabolic alkalosis uncompensated	Metabolic alkalosis with respiratory compensation
pH 7.52	pH 7.45
PaCO₂ 5.1	PaCO₂ 8.8
PaO₂ 10.5	PaO₂ 10.5
HCO₃ 38	HCO₃ 34
BE +12	BE +8

Table 3.11 A blood gas analysis algorithm.

(1) Look at pH: is it normal/acidotic/alkalotic?
  - If it is high, it is 'something' (either respiratory or metabolic) alkalosis.
  - If it is low, it is 'something' (either respiratory or metabolic) acidosis.
  - Determine the 'something' (either respiratory or metabolic) by looking at the other two parameters (PaCO₂ and HCO₃).
(2) Look at PaCO₂: is it normal/high/low?
  - If an acidosis or alkalosis is present as indicated by the pH, can it be accounted for by the PaCO₂?
  - Acidosis (low pH) is caused by high PaCO₂.
  - Alkalosis (high pH) is caused by low PaCO₂.
  - If the PaCO₂ is abnormal, the primary disorder is respiratory.
(3) Look at HCO₃/BE: is it normal/high/low?
  - If an acidosis or alkalosis is present as indicated by the pH and the PaCO₂ cannot account for it, can the HCO₃/BE levels account for it?
  - High HCO₃/BE levels indicate alkalosis.
  - Low HCO₃/BE levels indicate acidosis.
  - If the HCO₃/BE levels are abnormal, the primary disorder is metabolic.
(4) Once you have decided the primary disorder, look to see if there is any compensation.
  - Remember, in partial compensation, one parameter can account for the acidosis or alkalosis; the other parameter is going in the other direction to try to compensate.

pH but both the other parameters are abnormal, it is difficult to assess the primary disorder. Clinical patient information is required to help make this judgement.

Summary of ABG analysis

Table 3.11 shows a summary of a blood gas analysis algorithm.

CONTINUOUS INTRA-ARTERIAL BLOOD GAS MONITORING (CIBG)

Intermittent sampling of arterial blood may not detect rapid changes in the oxygenation, ventilation and acid–base status of critically ill children and infants and may also lead to iatrogenic hypovolaemia and anaemia in the very young from frequent sampling (Pakulla *et al.* 2004). Further, intermittent blood gas analysis is often performed after a clinical deterioration event (Menzel *et al.* 2003), as an ad hoc event or following a change in ventilator settings.

CIBG is used on very (level 3/4) critically ill (DH 1997) children (such as those with severe lung disease, those subjected to high-frequency oscillatory ventilation, nitric oxide or surfactant therapies, head-injured patients with raised intracranial pressure, shocked, septic or post-operative cardiac surgical patients (Weiss *et al.* 1999; Hatherill *et al.* 1997)) where continuous monitoring recognises changes early, permits immediate therapy alterations and monitors these. Further, it allows clinical decision-making to take into account trends rather than snap-shot values (MacIntosh & Britto 1999).

Other advantages include the potential for a reduction in the risk of infection due to the closed nature of the monitoring, the ability to detect responses to endotracheal suctioning and patient movement. It could be used in the development of improved weaning protocols with earlier extubation and therefore less ventilation time (MacIntosh & Britto 1999).

The catheter is often placed in the femoral artery, particularly in young children, but may also be placed in the radial artery (Weiss *et al.* 1999).

Check that:

- all values correlate with clinical assessment;
- the catheter/sensor does not have the potential to bend or kink;
- the line flushing fluid is adequate to prevent thrombus formation;
- the sensors are in the correct place and have not slipped into the flush solution (although the machine may provide an alert here);

- the sensors are not exposed to excess ambient light (e.g. lamps for heating) (although the machine may have an alert system for this);
- the waveform is adequate and demonstrates no signs of dampening down;
- the limb is continually assessed for warmth, pulses and capillary refill.

VENOUS BLOOD GAS SAMPLING

Blood gas analysis from sampling a vein can be useful in determining the adequacy of ventilatory status (PCO_2) and acid–base balance (pH). It provides information on oxygen consumption (VO_2) and ventilation status, but the results must be analysed in line with the patient's clinical condition. There appears to be good correlation between ABG analysis and both venous and capillary sampling, with the exception of the PO_2 value (Yildizdas *et al.* 2004).

Venous blood may be aspirated from:

(1) the pulmonary artery via the distal port of a pulmonary artery catheter.
- This technique is used in very (level 3/4) critically ill (DH 1997) children who have a pulmonary artery catheter inserted for haemodynamic monitoring (see Chapter 5).
- It is a highly risky procedure and should only be carried out by those health care professionals who have had the appropriate training.
- The mixed venous sample (SvO_2 – represents whole body venous blood) can reflect systemic perfusion and oxygen consumption (VO_2) values.
- A continuous saturation monitor (normal 65–75%) may be connected to the catheter to continually monitor data suggestive of cardiac output and oxygen uptake.
- Aspiration of the flushing fluid/fluid discard and sample must be made slowly to ensure sampling from the pulmonary capillary and not from across the capillary/alveolar interface.
- The catheter should then be flushed slowly to prevent clot formation within and at the distal end of the catheter.

(2) a peripheral catheter or puncture.
- This sample is less accurate in determining oxygen consumption.
- However, monitoring the pH/PCO_2 in this manner can give useful information on the patient's ventilation status and pH/HCO_3/BE can give useful information on the patient's metabolic status (as per arterial blood gas analysis above).
- This technique may be useful in a child or infant who does not require continuous monitoring via placement of an arterial catheter.
- It is less painful, has less risk of thrombosis and associated distal ischaemia and less chance of haemorrhage compared with arterial sampling (Yildizdas *et al.* 2004).

CAPILLARY BLOOD GAS SAMPLING

Blood gas analysis from sampling a capillary can be useful in determining the adequacy of respiratory function and acid–base balance. It provides information on ventilation status but the results must be analysed in line with the patient's clinical condition. There appears to be good correlation between ABG analysis and both venous and capillary sampling with the exception of the PO_2 value. However, the patient needs to be well perfused and therefore this technique is most useful in the mild to moderately ill child or infant (Yildizdas *et al.* 2004):

- The skin is usually punctured on the medial or lateral aspects of the heel in infants or the ear lobe and in one of the digits in toddlers and children (highly vascularised areas), as shown in Fig. 3.2.
- A blood glucose lancing device can be used to puncture the skin.
- The blood must be reasonably free-flowing and therefore good peripheral perfusion is required.
- It may be useful to warm the site to encourage good flow.
- This technique may be useful in a child who requires infrequent monitoring.

(AARC 1994)

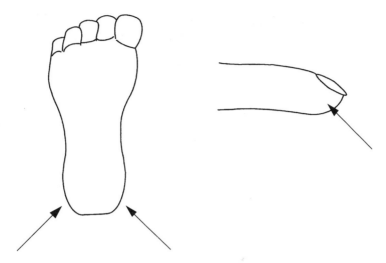

Fig. 3.2 Puncture sites for capillary blood gas sampling.

TRANSCUTANEOUS OXYGEN AND CARBON DIOXIDE BLOOD GAS MONITORING

Oxygenation and ventilation can be continuously monitored by estimating the partial pressure of oxygen ($PtcO_2$) and carbon dioxide ($PtcCO_2$), but the results must be analysed in line with the patient's clinical condition. $PtcO_2$ correlation with arterial blood gases is good if correctly used; however, $PtcCO_2$ is slightly less accurate. The skin is used to access the gases and therefore this method is best suited to the neonatal and young infant population.

The electrodes are attached to the skin surface and measure the diffusion of the gases through this semi-permeable membrane (Donn 2003). Current risk management training dictates that staff have the appropriately approved training to use the machine.

Attaching the electrodes
- Use water or saline to provide an adequate skin contact with the sensor.

- Ensure the electrodes are well stabilised with an adhesive ring.
- Heat the sensor to 43°C (immature infants with thin epithelium) or 44°C (larger infants with more developed and thicker epithelium), which causes the capillaries under the sensor to vasodilate, producing increased blood flow to the site (hyperaemia).
- Calibrate the sensors.
- Allow 10–15 minutes (or as per manufacturer's instructions) for an equilibration to ensure best accuracy.
- The membrane needs replacing on a frequent basis as part of ongoing maintenance.
- There may be a local protocol to regularly compare arterial blood sampling with transcutaneous readings for validation (AARC 2004).

(*Note your clinical area protocol here*:)

- Always consider the patient's clinical status with findings.
- Set high and low alarm settings.

Transcutaneous gas monitoring is useful:

- for monitoring ventilation and weaning processes;
- for assessing shunting by placing sensors on pre- and post-ductal sites (e.g. primary pulmonary hypertension of the newborn may be diagnosed and monitored) (AARC 2004);
- less often now as the use of pulse oximetry and capnography has increased.

Factors affecting accuracy (AARC 2004; Donn 2003) include:

- improper electrode placement or application;
- poor calibration;
- inaccurate low readings from:
  - poor perfusion states, e.g. acidosis, hypoxia, hypotension, shock
  - inadequate condition of site, e.g. bruising, oedema
  - hypothermia
  - shunting
  - pharmacological vaso-active agents, e.g. tolazoline.

Observe for the following potential complications (Donn 2003):

- areas of erythema from sensors sites: these usually resolve within 24 hours;
- blistering: change electrode position frequently, e.g. 2–4 hourly;
- thermal injury especially in extremely low birth weight (ELBW) infants or those infants with oedema and poor perfusion: change electrode position frequently, e.g. 2–4 hourly;
- damage to skin from adhesives: take care with removal.

END-TIDAL CARBON DIOXIDE (ETCO$_2$)/CAPNOGRAPHY

This monitoring system is useful in determining the patient's ventilation status by measuring carbon dioxide gases in expiration. The results must be analysed in line with the patient's clinical condition. The advantages (Curley & Thompson 2001) are that it:

- is non-invasive;
- has continuous monitoring;
- provides real time information.

With normal lung physiology and blood flow, ETCO$_2$ correlates well with PaCO$_2$ because ventilation (V) at the alveolar level is matched by perfusion (Q), but this correlation is greatly affected by many forms of pulmonary disease. Lung perfusion (blood flow) is required for the PaCO$_2$ to get to the alveolar-capillary membrane to enable the lungs to eliminate it. In cardiac arrest states or where there is ineffective lung perfusion (i.e. V/Q mismatching) and V/Q ratios are high (e.g. shock, pulmonary embolus), ETCO$_2$ will not reliably reflect PaCO$_2$ (Frakes 2001; Schallom & Ahrens 2001).

Hypoventilation and hyperventilation states are more likely to correlate with ETCO$_2$ results (Curley & Thompson 2001). However, using trends of the results rather than absolute values may be more clinically effective. Because of its need for tidal movements of air, ETCO$_2$ monitoring is ineffective with high frequency oscillatory ventilation (HFOV).

Other factors impacting on ETCO$_2$ other than ventilation include:

- fever
- pain
- shivering
- administration of sodium bicarbonate

$ETCO_2$ is measured in two ways (St. John 2003):

(1) Infrared spectroscopy: the exhaled gas is passed through infrared light. The amount of light absorbed is proportional to the concentration of carbon dioxide being exhaled. The result (capnometry) is expressed as:
  - a partial pressure (mmHg) of $PETCO_2$
  - a percentage (%) of carbon dioxide $ETCO_2$%.
(2) Colorimetric detection: the presence of carbon dioxide changes the pH-sensitive paper from purple to yellow. Results (capnometry) are only expressed as a colour.

Table 3.12 shows how $ETCO_2$ is measured using the different capnometers (machines) (Frakes 2001; St. John 2003).

False readings
High false readings may be due to the presence of water vapour and nitrous oxide; these absorb infrared light, giving higher readings (Frakes 2001). Low false readings may be due to an ETT leak or high oxygen concentrations being used; collisions between oxygen and carbon dioxide molecules change the infrared absorption of gas sample (Frakes 2001).

Indications for use of $ETCO_2$
- Monitoring of the critically ill child and infant (e.g. respiratory disease): may reduce the need for such frequent arterial blood gas analysis sampling.
- Monitoring the child with a head injury: continual monitoring may assist in prevention, early identification, and management of raised intracranial pressure due to raised $PaCO_2$.
- Helping determine the position of the endotracheal tube: $ETCO_2$ will not be evident from the stomach. However, bronchial migration may not be detected.
- Helping to determine an obstruction of the endotracheal tube by secretions or kinking of the tube.

Table 3.12 How ETCO$_2$ is measured using the different capnometers (machines).

Capnometer/ measure	Method	Clinical applications	Disadvantages
Sidestream Infrared spectroscopy	Exhaled gas is continually aspirated for samples	*Ventilated patients*: the device is placed in the side of the ventilator tubing *Non-ventilated patients*: the sampling tubing is placed near the patient's nares. Not always successful	Moisture and sputum may be drawn into the sample line: *ensure tubing remains clean and dry* Some devices are heavy: *support the device ensuring it is not pulling on the tubing* Child/infant may be intolerant or mouth-breathing or moving head away from sensor: *monitor patient*
Mainstream Infrared spectroscopy	Exhaled gas continually flows through the sensor	The device is placed within the exhalation ventilator tubing and is usually used on intubated patients	Some devices are heavy: *support the device, ensuring it is not pulling on the tubing* Increased deadspace
Disposable Colorimetric detection	Exhaled gas is exposed to pH-sensitive paper	Intubation of patients	No known disadvantages

- Providing an alarm if the patient becomes disconnected from the ventilator.
- Monitoring patients when weaning them from ventilatory support.
- Testing the placement of a naso-/oro-gastric tube: there is no carbon dioxide in the stomach.

(Curley & Thompson 2001; Frakes 2001; Schallom & Ahrens 2001)

4.5

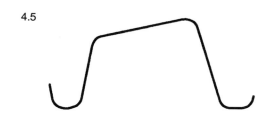

Fig. 3.3 A capnograph.

Capnography
This is the term used to define the value of the $ETCO_2$ and have it displayed graphically so that waveforms are recorded and analysed (Frakes 2001). Figure 3.3 shows a capnograph.

Capnogram
This is the characteristic waveform seen on the monitor. The carbon dioxide pressure is plotted against time and provides a breath-by-breath reading. $ETCO_2$ values should not be accepted without determining the quality of and analysing the waveform (Frakes 2001; St. John 2003). Table 3.13 shows capnogram analysis.

PEAK EXPIRATORY FLOW (PEF)
PEF is the greatest flow of air that can be produced during a forceful exhalation, usually occurring in the first fraction of a second of the exercise. It reflects the rate of flow from the large airways only. Airway obstruction will prolong the expiratory time and reduce the rate and volume of emptying, but in between bronchospasm episodes PEF may be normal. Usually children aged 5 years and over use this device (Campbell & McIntosh 1998) and their age, height, sex and race need to be taken into account when calculating normal values (Wong 1995). When monitoring a condition, trends may be just as important as the absolute values.

PEF is affected by:

- the co-operation of the child (including developmental ability);
- strength of the child's abdominal and thoracic muscles.

Table 3.13 Capnogram analysis.

Normal capnogram	Abnormal capnogram	Look for
During inspiration, there is no exhaled CO_2 so the waveform should be at baseline	*The baseline does not return to zero, i.e. on inspiration there is still CO_2 being sensed*	The patient has insufficient time for expiration The patient is rebreathing CO_2 There is insufficient inspiration
Even at the beginning of expiration, the gas will not contain much CO_2 as the anatomical deadspace is exhaled		
As exhalation commences and the air that has been involved in gas exchange is expired, the CO_2 pressure increases and is reflected in the sharp upstroke of the waveform	*The upstroke in expiration is at a less sharp angle, i.e. the expired air with the CO_2 is taking longer than usual to leave the lungs and reach the sensor*	The expiratory phase of respiration is being limited, e.g. occlusion or bronchospasm The endotracheal tube is kinked
The waveform plateaus with a slight upward stroke during this time of alveolar regional emptying NB: the digit $ETCO_2$ reading is taken at the end of this plateau	*The plateau is interrupted by a small dip, i.e. there is a small inspiration and expiration superimposed* *The plateau slope is shorter and slightly downwards, i.e. not all the alveoli are emptying*	The patient is spontaneously breathing when ventilated Hiccups The patient has bronchospasm
The waveform falls as exhalation ceases and inspiration washes the gas away from the sensor, this is reflected in the sharp downward deflection	*The downstroke at end-expiration/beginning inspiration is at a less sharp angle, i.e. inspiratory gas is not washing the $ETCO_2$ away from the sensor quickly enough*	A leak in the ventilator system, around the endotracheal tube or in the endotracheal tube cuff
	Loss of waveform/waveform near baseline	Ventilator disconnection Endotracheal tube displacement or obstruction Equipment malfunction
	Change of $ETCO_2$ reading but consistent waveform	A change in ventilation parameters or cardiac output A change in ventilation tubing, size or position

PEF can provide an objective and reproducible method of evaluating the presence and degree of lung disease (often asthma) as well as the response to therapy (e.g. bronchodilators) (Wong 1995):

- at home to monitor condition;
- at school to assist with decision-making;
- at the GP clinic to monitor condition/measure response to therapy;
- in the Emergency Department or in-patient ward to measure response to therapy.

PEF can be measured using:

- a pneumotachometer, which uses a transducer to convert the flow to an electrical signal during spirometry; or
- a simple portable flow gauge, a rapid, adaptable, portable device; a marker within the device is pushed along a scale and comes to rest at a point measuring PEF.

The PEF manoeuvre may include consideration of:

- asking the child to stand;
- asking the child to hold/the practitioner to hold the meter lightly;
- ensuring that the flow meter is set at zero;
- ensuring that fingers do not get in the way of the marker;
- asking the child to take a deep breath;
- opening the mouth and closing the lips around the mouthpiece, holding it horizontally;
- blowing hard and fast, asking the child to produce the biggest 'huff' he/she can;
- three attempts to measure the best effort (Campbell & McIntosh 1998);
- documentation including the percentage of any inhaled oxygen or therapy (e.g. bronchodilators).

The use of PEF monitoring in children has been challenged by expert practitioners and other respiratory monitoring, e.g. forced expiratory volume in one second (FEV1) may be used as an alternative (Eid *et al.* 2000).

CHEST X-RAY INTERPRETATION

The chest X-ray is the most commonly performed paediatric radiological investigation (Arthur 2000). The process of interpreting the findings must include the age of the child, the clinical history and examination and any other laboratory findings. It is also important to understand the differing anatomy of the developing infant and child (Beckstrand 2001). The basic principles (Beckstrand 2001) are outlined below:

- X-rays are a form of short wavelength radiant energy (part of the electromagnetic spectrum) produced by the X-ray tube.
- The film, image or radiograph is the result that is interpreted.
- The radiograph is produced when X-rays are passed through the body to the photosensitive cassette (Arthur 2000; Beckstrand 2001). Table 3.14 shows different radiograph views.
- Those body structures that are very dense (e.g. metal, bone or catheters) block most of the rays, preventing them from reaching the film, and produce a white or radio opaque image.
- Tissue and water (diaphragm, heart, thymus, great vessels) block the rays less effectively and produce a grey image.
- X-rays easily travel through less dense structures (e.g. air in lungs or stomach) to the film and produce a more radio lucent or dark grey/black image.
- Hence, radiology is the science of interpreting different densities.
- When structures with different densities are adjacent, they produce contrasting silhouettes (e.g. the heart can easily be seen against a normal lung field).
- It is difficult to distinguish organs lying together that have similar densities (e.g. thymus and heart), resulting in a silhouette (e.g. cardiothymic silhouette).
- The density can be changed by a disease process, which will be reflected in the X-ray film:
  - for example, if atelectasis develops, the lung takes on a more water-like density and the film becomes more opaque;

Table 3.14 Radiograph views.

View	Explanation	Advantages and disadvantages
Postero-anterior (PA)	For the ambulant older child who can stand or sit Usually performed within the radiology department The X-rays pass from the posterior chest through to the anterior The film plate is positioned anteriorly to the patient's chest The sick child may be positioned prone	Provides the best quality film Positioning of the arms moves the shoulder blades laterally and displaces the scapulas, providing good lung visual Heart shadow is more accurate in size Horizontal fluid levels (e.g. stomach or pleura) are readily apparent
Antero-posterior (AP) – erect	For the sick child who cannot leave his/her bed but can sit upright Usually performed at the bedside with a portable X-ray machine The X-rays pass from the anterior chest through to the posterior The film plate is placed behind the patient's back	Heart is further away and therefore appears slightly larger due to magnification Mediastinal width *may* also be exaggerated Horizontal fluid levels (e.g. stomach or pleura) are readily apparent
Antero-posterior (AP) – supine	For those who cannot sit up or stand including children who are critically ill and infants Performed at the bedside with a portable X-ray machine The X-rays pass from the anterior chest through to the posterior The film plate is placed behind the patient's back	Pleural fluid and pneumothoraces are more difficult to detect Gastric air bubble may be less apparent as any fluid may 'level out'
Lateral – erect or supine	The film plate is placed on the left or right side of the patient's chest	Demonstrates air/fluid levels
Oblique	The exposure of the X-rays is angled and may be appropriate for suspected spondylosis, especially in recruits or young athletes (gymnasts, wrestlers)	Usually produces an increase in radiation exposure
Lordotic	Occurs when a supine view is being attempted The abdomen is higher than the chest and shoulders The X-rays are delivered at an angle Usually occurs in infants who are trying to wriggle away from the X-ray plate Can easily occur when infants are ventilated if their heads are turned to one side and the weight and tension of the ventilator tubing causes the opposite shoulder to lift	Interpretation of anatomy and position of catheters is severely limited Reducing the risk may include: – warming the cassette – placing cassette under warm, light blanket – raising head of bed 5–10° – tilting the X-ray tube 5–10° towards the feet – allowing the infant a short time to adjust and quieten

o the patient will also lose his or her contrasting heart borders, as the heart has a water-like density, similar to the atelectic areas of the lung.

Radiation exposure (Trotter & Carey 2000)

Patients should have X-rays only when clinically indicated. Further, precautions must be considered to limit X-ray exposure:

- Gonad protection should be instituted.
- All staff should remain at a minimum of 2 m away from the exposure.
- A lead apron must be used if patient contact is required during the procedure (do not undertake if pregnant).

The X-ray film: what are you looking at (Arthur 2000; Trotter & Carey 2000; Beckstrand 2001)?

(1) Correct labelling
  - Check patient's name and date of the X-ray investigation.
  - Check the film is placed on the viewing board with the 'L' (patient's left side) or 'R' (patient's right side) correctly positioned. Dextrocardia or lung pathology distorting the lungs will be seen as a right-sided heart on the X-ray film.
  - Check the projection (PA or AP/supine or erect).
(2) Quality of the film
  - Look at the exposure of the film. Correct exposure provides some visibility of the vertebral column through the cardiac shadow and clear pulmonary vasculature markings.
  - If the film is too dark, it has been overexposed and the normal contrast between the lung fields and film background has been lost; few lung markings can be seen.
  - An underexposed film appears much lighter than normal or hazy and the spinal column cannot be seen through the heart shadow.
(3) Position, rotation and symmetry
  - Shoulders, chest or body rotation on the film will distort the features and limit interpretation.

- Check:
  - the spine is lying in the middle of the chest; clavicles are equidistant;
  - symmetry of each hemi-thorax by comparing one lung field to the other;
  - the ribs on each side are similar in length;
  - that the diaphragm compares bilaterally.
- Check for lordosis:
  - the upper, posterior ribs may appear more horizontal;
  - the anterior ribs may appear more 'upturned' and higher than the posterior ribs;
  - the endotracheal tube may appear high;
  - the heart may appear boot-shaped.
- Check for flexed head:
  - the upper zones of the lungs may be masked;
  - the endotracheal tube may be high.
- Check for extended head:
  - the endotracheal tube may be low.

(4) Phase of respiration
- Good inspiration is required for effective interpretation.
- An expiratory film may show hazy lung fields, enlarged heart and enhanced broncho-vesicular markings, all potentially leading to misdiagnosis.
- Check there are 5–7 (child) and 8–9 (infant) anterior ribs above the right diaphragm (the left is lower).

(5) Artefacts
- These need to be recognised so that they are not mistaken for pathology. The X-ray film can also be used to verify the placement of catheters and tubes inserted to assist with patient management.
- Consider the following:
  - vertical skin folds in premature infants may simulate a pneumothorax;
  - plaited hair, jewellery or ornaments will project over the lung fields and mediastinum;
  - monitoring leads may cover relatively large portions of the chest (it is preferable to remove these prior to X-ray

if appropriate or place ECG dots on child's shoulders);

o the position of the endotracheal tube:
  – the tube should sit approximately 2 cm above the level of the carina;
  – or the tip of the ETT should be at the level of T2–T4;

o the naso-/oro-gastric tube: the tube may be followed from the mouth down the oesophagus and into the stomach. It may curl once inside the stomach. The presence of gas may be elucidated;

o chest tubes: drains may be placed in the pleura to drain air, blood, chyle or pus or the mediastinum to drain blood post cardiac surgery;

o pacing wires: these are usually placed during heart surgery. They may be seen curled up as they are secured to the chest or trailing if attached to a pacing box;

o permanent pacing boxes may be determined depending on where they have been placed;

o central venous catheters may be placed in the jugular vein, subclavian vein or umbilical vein: their position can be determined on the X-ray plate;

o pulmonary artery catheters can be traced to determine correct positioning;

o artificial valves and placement of cardiac shunt may also be seen.

(6) Bony framework
  • Check for equality, size, number and continuity of:
    o clavicles
    o ribs: are more horizontal in infants
    o vertebrae

(7) Trachea
  • Check for air column and deviation.

(8) Bronchi and hilum
  • The hilum is the area to the left and right of the heart borders and includes the bronchi, pulmonary vessels and nerves.

- Check for vascular appearances in the proximal two-thirds of the lung.

(9) Mediastinum
- Check for a clear heart border.
- Determine the cardio-thoracic ratio: the heart should occupy no more than 60% of the thoracic cage in the infant and 50% in the child (in an AP X-ray).
- The thymus gland is a large but variable sized structure in infants, getting smaller in comparison in the child. It is seen as a mass that merges discretely on the superior heart shadow.
- Older girls' X-ray films may show mammary glands.

(10) Diaphragm
- The right hemi diaphragm may be slightly higher than the left because of the positioning of the heart.
- Check that they look even.
- There may be air under the left diaphragm, indicating air in the stomach.

(11) Lung fields
- There should be no vascular appearances in outer lung fields.
- Check for a uniform radiolucent appearance except in hilar and perihilar regions.
- A particular pattern throughout all lung fields is referred to as 'diffuse, homogenous or symmetrical'.
- Look for areas of more density, indicating pathology.
- Determine if the changes are inside or outside the lung:
  - inside the lung, the 'whiteness' or opaqueness may indicate that a fluid-like density pathology is developing, e.g. atelectasis;
  - outside the lung, in pleura, medistinum or pericardial spaces
    - the 'whiteness' or opaqueness may indicate that a fluid-like density pathology is replacing the air, e.g. pleural effusion
    - the 'blackness' or lucency may indicate that an air-like density pathology has developed, e.g. pneumothorax.

APNOEA MONITORS (MATTRESS)

Apnoea monitors are mostly used in the home to continually track the respiratory rate (with or without the heart rate) of the infant. Some machines will have facilities to download specific episodes. Apnoeas of infancy or prematurity are unexplained episodes of cessation of breathing for more than 20 seconds or one that is accompanied by circulatory compromise, e.g. pallor, bradycardia, hypotonia. Families who are advised to use home apnoea monitoring are given the appropriate training in cardio-pulmonary resuscitation and use of the equipment.

Note:

- Check the manufacturer's instructions for placement of the pad, e.g. it may be placed under the mattress rather than the infant's body.
- The apnoea mattress has a pressure-sensitive pad that detects the change in weight distribution that occurs during respiration.
- The sensor may fail to detect an obstructive or mixed apnoea due to the continuing movement of the infant's chest.
- During apnoea associated with a bradycardia, the cardiac impulse may increase in intensity which can prevent the alarm from sounding if the sensitivity of the alarm is too high.
- Check the monitor frequently to ensure it is working, including electrical and battery supply.
- Adhesive electrodes or a belt with electrodes attached are used when heart rate is also monitored.

SUMMARY

There are a range of technological adjuncts assisting the health care practitioner to assess and monitor the respiratory system. The results must be interpreted in conjunction with physical examination and the patient's condition. Adequate training is required to use the technology safely and accurately.

REFERENCES

American Association for Respiratory Care (AARC) (1994) AARC clinical practice guideline; capillary blood gas sampling for neonatal and pediatric patients. *Respiratory Care*, **39** (12), 1180–1183.

American Association for Respiratory Care (AARC) (2004) AARC clinical practice guideline; transcutaneous blood gas monitoring for neonatal and pediatric patients. *Respiratory Care*, **49** (9), 1069–1072.

Arthur, R. (2000) Interpretation of the paediatric chest x-ray. *Paediatric Respiratory Reviews*, **1**, 41–50.

Beaumont, T. (1997) How to guides: arterial blood gas sampling. *Care of the Critically Ill*, **13** (1), centre insert.

Beckstrand, R.L. (2001) Understanding chest radiographs of infants and children: the AIR systematic approach. *Critical Care Nurse*, **21** (3), 54–65.

Bohnhorst, B., Peter, C.S. & Poets, C.F. (2002) Detection of hyperoxaemia in neonates: data from three new pulse oximeters. *Archives of Disease in Childhood*, **87** (3), 217–220.

Campbell, A.G.M. & McIntosh, N. (1998) *Forfar and Arneil's Textbook of Pediatrics*, 5th edn. Churchill Livingston, New York.

Chandler, T. (2000) Oxygen saturation monitoring. *Paediatric Nursing*, **12** (8), 37–42.

Coté, C.J., Goldstein, A., Fuchsman, W.H. & Hoaglin, D.C. (1988) The effect of nail polish on pulse oximetry. *Anesthesia and Analgesia*, **67**, 683–686.

Curley, M.A.Q. & Moloney-Harmon, P.A. (eds) *Critical Care Nursing of Infants and Children*, 2nd edn. W.B. Saunders, Philadelphia.

Curley, M.A.Q. & Thompson, J.E. (2001) Oxygenation and ventilation. Acid–base balance. In: Curley, M.A.Q. & Moloney-Harmon, P.A. (eds) *Critical Care Nursing of Infants and Children*, 2nd edn. W.B. Saunders, Philadelphia, pp 309–321.

Department of Health (1997) *Paediatric Intensive Care: A Framework for the Future*. NHS Executive, Department of Health, London.

Eid, N., Yandell, B., Howell, L., Eddy, M. & Sheikh, S. (2000) Can peak expiratory flow predict airflow obstruction in children with asthma? *Pediatrics*, **105** (2), 354–358.

Frakes, M.A. (2001) Measuring end-tidal carbon dioxide: clinical applications and usefulness. *Critical Care Nurse*, **21** (5), 23–37.

Grap, M.J. (2002) Protocols for practice. Applying research at the bedside. Pulse oximetry. *Critical Care Nurse*, **22** (3), 69–73.

Hatherill, M., Tibby, S.M., Durward, A., Rajah, V. & Murdoch, I.A. (1997) Continuous intra-arterial blood-gas monitoring in infants and children with cyanotic heart disease. *British Journal of Anaesthesia*, **79**, 665–667.

Jevon, P. & Ewens, B. (2002) *Monitoring the Critically Ill Patient.* Blackwell Science, Oxford.

MacIntosh, I. & Britto, J. (1999) How to guide: continuous intra-arterial blood gas monitoring. *Care of the Critically Ill,* **15** (3), centre insert.

Martin, L. (1999) *All You Really Need To Know to Interpret Arterial Blood Gases.* Lippincott, Williams and Wilkins, Philadelphia.

Menzel, M., Soukup, J., Henze, D., *et al.* (2003) Experiences with continuous intra-arterial blood gas monitoring: precision and drift of a pure optode-system. *Intensive Care Medicine,* **29** (2), 2180–2186.

Milner, A. & Hull, D. (1998) *Hospital Pediatrics,* 3rd edn. Churchill Livingston, London.

Moyle, J. (1999) Pulse oximetry. *Journal of Neonatal Nursing,* **5** (2), insert 4 pp.

Pakulla, M.A., Obal, D. & Loer, S.A. (2004) Continuous intra-arterial blood gas monitoring in rats. *Laboratory Animals,* **38**, 133–137.

Royal Children's Hospital (RCH) (2003) *Neonatal Handbook: Blood Gas Interpretation.* http://www.rch.org.au/nets/handbook, accessed 12/10/04.

Sado, D.M. & Deakin, C.D. (2005) Local anaesthesia for venous cannulation and arterial blood gas sampling: are doctors using it? *Journal of the Royal Society of Medicine,* **98** (4), 158.

Schallom, L. & Ahrens, T. (2001) Hemodynamic applications of capnography. *Journal of Cardiovascular Nursing,* **15** (2), 56–70.

Sheehy, S. & Lombardi, J. (1995) *Emergency Care,* 4th edn. Mosby, St. Louis.

Simpson, H. (2004) Interpretation of arterial blood gases: a clinical guide for nurses. *British Journal of Nursing,* **13** (9), 522–528.

Slota, M. (1998) *American Association of Critical Care Nurses: Core Curriculum for Pediatric Critical Care Nursing.* W.B. Saunders, Philadelphia.

Smith, T. (1995) Pulse oximetry. *Journal of Neonatal and Paediatric Critical Care,* **1** (3), 5–18.

Steele, A. (1999) Allen's test is not routinely used before a radial arterial puncture. *British Medical Journal,* **318**, 734.

St. John, R.E. (2003) End-tidal carbon dioxide monitoring. *Critical Care Nurse,* **23** (4), 83–88.

Trotter, C. & Carey, B.E. (2000) Radiology basics: overview and concepts. *Neonatal Network,* **19** (2), 35–47.

Weiss, I.K., Fink, S., Harrison, R., Feldman, D. & Brill, J.E. (1999) Clinical use of continuous arterial blood gas monitoring in the pediatric intensive care unit. *Pediatrics,* **103** (2), 440–445.

Wong, D. (1995) *Whaley and Wong's Nursing Care of Infants and Children,* 5th edn. Mosby, St Louis.

Woodrow, P. (2004) Arterial blood gas analysis. *Nursing Standard*, **18** (21), 45–52.

Yildizdas, D., Yapicioglu, H.L., Yilmaz, H.L. & Sertdemir, Y. (2004) Correlation of simultaneously obtained capillary, venous, and arterial blood gases of patients in a paediatric intensive care unit. *Archives of Disease in Childhood*, **89**, 176–180.

Cardiovascular Assessment

4

INTRODUCTION

Cardiovascular examination in infants and children is an important aspect of assessment in the sick child or the child preparing for treatment, including surgery and drug therapy. Also, congenital heart disease (CHD) is the most common of congenital anomalies and therefore history-taking and examination are essential (Archer & Birch 1998).

Physical examination of the cardiovascular system utilises the skills of inspection, palpation and auscultation. Although the text is set out using this format, practitioners will develop their own technique in combining aspects of the examination. However, it has been recommended that auscultation is left until the end (Gill & O'Brien 2002). There is a close association with the respiratory system (e.g. colour, clubbing, mottling, respiratory difficulty and level of consciousness), but only those points pertinent specifically to cardiovascular examination are presented here. It is worth noting that the infant in respiratory distress does not automatically have a respiratory cause for it. This chapter is divided into two: the cardiac and the peripheral vascular systems. The aim of this chapter is to understand the principles of cardiac and peripheral vascular examination for different ages.

LEARNING OBJECTIVES

By the end of this chapter the reader will be able to:

❑ Appreciate the importance of taking a history.
❑ Outline the steps of a comprehensive assessment.
❑ Recognise symptoms of cardiac failure and shock.

HISTORY
A comprehensive history provides a significant amount of information, and information about the pregnancy and post-natal status is also required (see Chapter 1). Other specific aspects include:

- respiratory symptoms/infections;
- difficulty in feeding in infants (there is a great metabolic demand during feeding and a rapid respiratory rate decreases time for swallowing);
- failure to thrive and poor weight gain in infants (may be made worse by increased caloric needs of overworked myocardium);
- increased sympathetic activity causes excessive perspiration;
- fatigue;
- decreased tolerance for exercise;
- weakness;
- oedema in older infants and children
- dizziness
- epistaxis;
- spelling (an hypoxic event where the infundibulum of the right ventricular outflow track contracts/spasms and causes loss of blood flow to the lungs; the patient will become very cyanosed and may lose consciousness; may be seen in tetralogy of Fallot);
- squatting (see under 'Inspection' below);
- previous heart surgery.

PHYSICAL ASSESSMENT
Whilst maintaining adequate dignity and privacy, the child's chest and extremities at times need to be naked for effective examination. It may be appropriate to ask teenage girls to displace their breasts for examination if necessary.

VITAL SIGNS
The pulse
As systole and diastole occur within the cardiac cycle, the arterial wall distends and then recoils, causing the pulse. All pulses

should be evaluated and compared (see under 'Palpation'). The pulse needs to be evaluated for rate, rhythm and volume.

Rate

- Rate is related to age and activity, with variations brought on by distress, fever (there can be an increase of up to 10 beats per degree increase in temperature), excitement and exercise. Table 4.1 shows normal values of pulse rate for different age groups (Curley & Moloney-Harmon 2001).
- Auscultating the apex is the most accurate way of counting heart rate in infants (Sarti *et al.* 2005).
- The brachial pulse is also useful for evaluation in infants. It can be found just above the cubital fossa.
- The radial pulse is palpated in the over 2 years old age group.
- Counting should be taken over a 30-second period if normal and a full minute if any abnormalities are detected (Horrox 2002).

Rhythm

- Sinus arrhythmia is normal and commonly found in children. The rate increases slightly on inspiration and decreases on expiration (Campbell & McIntosh 1998).
- For any irregularity, evaluate how regular the irregularity is.

Volume

- Volume is usually assessed as (1) weak, (2) normal or (3) bounding.

Table 4.1 Pulse rate normal values.

Age	Pulse rate range (asleep → awake)
Newborn/infant	80–160
Toddler/pre-schooler	60–110
School age	60–110
Young person	50–90

- Full volume pulses are produced from:
  - lesions with a wide pulse pressure (difference between systolic and diastolic);
  - lesions causing shunting, e.g. ventricular septal defect or patent ductus arteriosus (Gill & O'Brien 2002);
  - warm shocked state (e.g. sepsis);
- Thready, weak or small volume pulses are indicative of hypotension/impending shock (cold shock)/heart failure.

Blood pressure
(Basic skill)
- Blood pressure may be defined as cardiac output × systemic vascular resistance.
- It should always be measured as part of the examination.
- Children have the ability to compensate well to a decreased cardiac output (vasoconstriction, tachycardia and increased myocardial contractility), so a finding of hypotension is a late sign of decompensated shock that requires immediate life support resuscitation (Resuscitation Council (UK) 2004).
- The systolic blood pressure value is caused by the force of the contraction of the left ventricle and blood ejected into the arterial vessels.
- The diastole value reflects the recoil of the artery and relaxation of the heart.
- The mean arterial pressure (MAP) value provides information on the perfusion to the coronary arteries, organs and peripheral capillary bed.
- MAP = 1/3 systolic + 2/3 diastolic.
- Repeating the measurement two to three times with short intervals may be required to get an accurate result. Table 4.2 shows normal blood pressure ranges for different age groups.

Techniques
The following techniques are used to check blood pressure:

(1) Sphygmomanometer (listening for Korotkoff's sounds made when blood returns to the artery after compression):
  - may be more useful in the older child;

Table 4.2 Normal blood pressure ranges (Resuscitation Council (UK) 2004).

Age	Systolic	Diastolic	Mean
Premature: less than 1 kg	39–59	16–36	24–43
Newborn: 3 kg	50–70	25–45	33–53
Newborn: 4 days	60–90	20–60	33–70
Infant: 6 months	87–105	53–66	64–79
Child: 2 years	95–105	53–66	67–79
Child: 7 years	97–112	57–71	70–84
Young person	112–128	66–80	81–96

- keep arm, heart and sphygmomanometer on same horizontal plane, as gravity may distort reading.
(2) Oscillometry (machine detects the vibrations that occur when blood returns to the artery after compression), e.g. Dinamap:
    - may be more useful in the younger child and infant.
(3) Invasive arterial monitoring: see under 'Haemodynamic Monitoring' (Chapter 5).

Obtaining accurate results
In order to maximise the opportunity for an accurate result (Park & Menard 1987):

- use the right arm (using the thigh may give a false high reading);
- compare with left arm and at least one leg if coarctation of the aorta is suspected; often the blood pressure of all four limbs is taken (use appropriate-size cuffs for arms and legs);
- have the child seated, standing or lying down;
- use diversion techniques to keep the child's anxiety levels low;
- use the correct-size cuff with a bladder that completely encircles the arm:
    - for infants and small children use a cuff that covers almost the full length of the upper arm when the arm is bent (Roy 1997);

o for older children, use a cuff that covers two thirds of the upper arm.

Using the sphygmomanometer (Jowett 1997)
(1) Find the brachial artery and monitor it with fingertips.
(2) Blow up the cuff until the pulse disappears and note the related sphygmomanometer pressure.
(3) Let the cuff down completely.
(4) Place the diaphragm of the stethoscope over the brachial artery.
(5) Blow up the cuff to a slightly higher level than the related sphygmomanometer pressure estimated above.
(6) Release the cuff slowly at no more than 2–3 mmHg/second.
(7) Have the sphygmomanometer at eye level and observe the pressure falling.
(8) Note when the first Korotkoff's sounds (phase 1) are heard. This represents systole.
(9) The sound will disappear (phase 2).
(10) The sound will return (phase 3).
(11) The sounds become faint (phase 4) This represents diastole blood pressure in the child under 12 years old.
(12) The sound completely disappears again (phase 5). This represents diastolic blood pressure in the child over 12 years old.

Document
The following should be documented:

- technique of measurement
- size of cuff
- limb used
- position of the child
- anxiety state of the child

Inaccurate readings
Inaccurate readings may occur due to:

- obesity
- atrial flutter or fibrillation
- a cuff too small (gives a false high reading) (Roy 1997)

- a cuff too large (gives a false low reading)
- perished equipment

Pulsus paradoxus
(Advanced skill)
The normal systolic blood pressure may decrease up to 8 mmHg during normal inspiration and even more during deep inspiration. Pulsus paradoxus exists when the blood pressure decreases more than this. The technique is as follows:

- Blow up the cuff until no Karotkoff sounds are heard.
- Observe the child's respirations.
- Slowly deflate the cuff and note the pressure when the Karotkoff sounds disappear on inspiration and then expiration.

This is not an easy activity to undertake and you will need to decide the clinical significance of undertaking this aspect of assessment.

Pulsus paradoxus occurs in respiratory (asthma, emphysema) and cardiac (cardiac tamponade, effusion, hypovolaemia) disorders (Bickley 2003) and is an ominous sign.

Pulsus alternans
(Advanced skill)
In pulsus alternans the systolic blood pressure is alternately high and low. It is indicative of left ventricular failure.

CARDIAC ASSESSMENT
Inspection
Anterior chest
(Basic skill)
Examine the chest from an angle as well as directly; this may help identify findings. Look at:

(1) The skin:
   - for any scarring that may indicate thoracic surgery or trauma.
(2) The precordium (the chest):
   - for any obvious bulging (the sternum and ribs bow forwards, giving the chest an overblown appearance) that may indicate chronic heart enlargement.

(3) The left and right lower sternal borders/xiphisternum (infants have a right ventricular muscle mass that is greater than the left ventricle; thus right ventricular dominance is seen in neonates/young infants, gradually being replaced by left ventricular dominance as the child grows):
- for (1) a right ventricular (RV) impulse, or (2) diffuse heaves or lifts that might indicate RV enlargement.

(4) The apical area:
- for (1) a left ventricular (LV) impulse; this is frequently seen in the thin child, in a child with a hyperdynamic status (fever, excitement) or in a child with true LV enlargement (Gill & O'Brien 2002), or (2) diffuse heaves or lifts that might indicate LV enlargement.

Jugular venous pressure (JVP)

(Advanced skill)

This examination is difficult to undertake in the child, particularly infants and young children who have short, stocky necks and may have prominent external jugular veins (Archer & Birch 1998). It is therefore mainly used in children over 12 years of age. See Fig. 4.1 for landmarks.

The technique is as follows:

- The young person lies on the bed with a pillow under the head.
- Raise the head of the bed 30°.
- Turn the young person's head away from the side you are inspecting (usually the patient's right side).
- Identify the external jugular vein.
- Identify the internal jugular pulsations (the internal jugular vein lies deep in the sternomastoid muscles and is not palpable but pulsations are visible)
  - in the suprasternal notch
  - between where the sternomastoid muscles attach to the sternum and clavicle
- Identify the highest point of the internal jugular pulsations.
- Place a ruler vertically from the sternal angle.
- Use a card or ruler to connect from the pulsations to the vertical ruler.

- Note where the card intersects the vertical ruler.
- This is the jugular venous pressure as measured in centimetres.

Note:

- A value less than 5 cm is normal; greater than this can indicate right heart failure.
- If the patient is hypovolaemic, he/she may need to lie flat before the pulsations are visible.
- With increased JVP, the patient may need to sit up at a greater angle before the pulsations can be seen.
- Always document at which angle the patient was lying when recording findings.

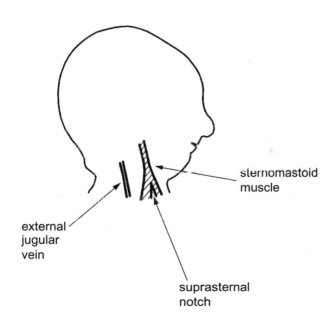

Fig. 4.1 Landmarks for measuring jugular venous pressure.

Palpation
(Advanced skill)
Palpation is performed in order to:

- confirm and qualify visible findings;
- detect other normal and abnormal findings.

Fingertips are usually used for detecting pulsations, but in infants it may be easier to use the base of the fingers. Use the ball of the hand or side of the hand for detecting vibratory thrills or rubs. Vibratory thrills are produced by the flow of blood from one chamber to another through a narrowed or abnormal opening (e.g. a stenotic valve or a septal defect). They can feel like the belly of a purring cat and are best detected during expiration (Engel 1997).

Precordium

(1) Palpate all over the precordium for pulsations and thrills:
- a thrill in the suprasternal notch may suggest coarctation of the aorta or aortic stenosis (Gill & O'Brien 2002);
- right ventricular enlargement may be determined by a forceful pulsation or thrill, palpated along the left and right sternal edges or to the left and right of the xiphisternum in neonates/young infants (Roy 1997). Infants have a right ventricular muscle mass that is greater than the left ventricle; thus right ventricular dominance is seen in infants, gradually being replaced by left ventricular dominance as the child grows.
(2) Identify the apical impulse (also called the point of maximal impulse or PMI); this is the impulse felt when the left ventricle contracts and touches the chest wall:
- in infants and young children, this is found in the midclavicular line at the level of the 4th intercostal space (one space higher than adults due to the heart lying more horizontally in the chest) (Bickley 2003);
- in older children, it is found in the midclavicular line at the level of the 5th intercostal space;
- it is difficult to find in plump and healthy infants (especially if they have a full stomach) but, overall, the chest wall of children is thin and it should be detectable;

- a diffuse, forceful and displaced (lateral) apex may indicate LV hypertrophy but may also indicate a hyperdynamic state, e.g. anaemia, fever or anxiety.

Auscultation
- In infants and children, where heart rates are high, this technique is difficult to carry out. It requires concentration and practice; minimise any environmental noise and use pacifiers or distraction techniques in the infant and younger child.
- Know in advance the normal sounds and where they are heard.
- The respiratory sounds and a crying infant also add to the difficulty in distinguishing heart sounds. It may be helpful, on occasions, to blow a puff of air into the face of infants. This usually causes them to cease breathing for a few seconds (Roy 1997).
- Both the diaphragm and bell are required to hear both high-pitched and low-pitched sounds respectively.
- Examination should take place with the child sitting and lying, as some signs can disappear on sitting.

The areas for auscultation are located in the direction of blood flow through the cardiac valves. Figure 4.2 shows the cardiac areas.

Normal heart sounds (Jordan & Scott 1989)
(Basic skill)
S1:

- The first heart sound ('lubb') is heard loudest at the mitral or apical area.
- It is longer and lower pitched than S2.
- It represents the closure of the atrio-ventricular valves; the mitral and tricuspid valves are forced shut at the beginning of contraction.
- It is normally heard with the diaphragm, but the bell can also be used (Gill & O'Brien 2002).
- This sound is synchronous with peripheral pulses.
- The sound may be split and may be heard at the tricuspid area where the tricuspid valve is closing slightly later than the mitral valve (normal finding in children).

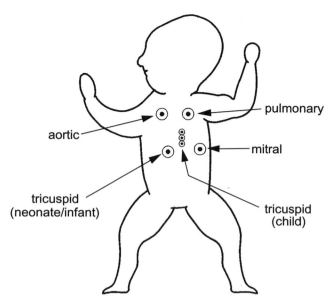

Fig. 4.2 Cardiac areas.

S2:

- The second heart sound ('dubb') is best heard at the aortic area.
- It represents closure of semi-lunar valves; the aortic and pulmonary valves are forced to close at the beginning of diastole.
- The sound is short and high pitched (use diaphragm).
- It may be split during inspiration (physiological split) and may be accentuated if the breath is held on inspiration.
- The split sound may be heard best at the pulmonary area where the pulmonary valve is closing slightly later than the aortic valve (Roy 1997).

Evaluate sounds for (Bickley 2003):

- quality: are they clear and distinct?
- rate: are they synchronous with the pulse?

- intensity: are they consistent with what would normally be found?
- rhythm: are they regular?

Additional heart sounds
(Advanced skill)

S3:

- The third heart sound is usually normal in infants and young children.
- It is produced as a result of the vibrations caused during the high flow filling of the ventricles.
- It is heard early in diastole, just after S2, over the ventricle in which they occur.
- The sound is dull and low pitched (use bell).

S4:

- The fourth heart sound is an abnormal finding.
- It is caused by resistance to ventricular filling following atrial contraction and is indicative of a poorly compliant ventricle.
- It is heard at the end of diastole just before S1.
- It is low pitched (use bell).

S3 and S4 *may* best be heard with the child lying on his or her left side.

Ejection click
(Advanced skill)

- This abnormal sound reflects the beginning of the ejection of blood into a dilated great vessel.
- It is usually associated with abnormalities of the opening of the pulmonary or aortic valve.
- It is a high pitched sound (use diaphragm).
- It is usually heard just after S1.

Opening snap
(Advanced skill)

- This sound reflects the mitral or tricuspid valve opening and the commencement of diastolic flow into the ventricles.
- It is a high pitched sound (use diaphragm).

- It is heard loudest over respective valves.
- It is heard immediately after S2 and before S3.

A 'gallop rhythm' usually indicates a triple rhythm including a combination of S1, S2 and a third sound, e.g. S3, S4 or a click (Roy 1997).

Murmurs
(Advanced skill)
- These are difficult to hear as the examiner has to try to dismiss all extraneous sounds and listen between heart sounds for murmurs.
- Take plenty of time to try to evaluate these sounds (Archer & Birch 1998).
- They are caused by either turbulence in the blood or tissue vibration.
- They are longer in duration in comparison to the heart sounds above.
- See Table 4.3 for evaluation of murmurs.

Distinguishing between innocent and pathologic murmurs is challenging. Table 4.4 shows the differences. Table 4.5 shows the characteristics of some common murmurs (Engel 1997; Archer & Birch 1998).

Friction rubs
(Advanced skill)
- Friction rubs produce a scratchy high-pitched grating sound (use diaphragm).
- Usually they occur when two membranes are inflamed and rub together, e.g. in the pleural or pericardial sac.
- Pleural rubs cease with breath holding. This may be a helpful distinguishing feature in the co-operative child.

Bruits
(Advanced skill)
- These sounds are murmur-like but occur in arteries. They are palpated as thrills and auscultated as bruits.
- Determine where they fall in the cardiac cycle.
- Pre-school age children and young school-age children may have an innocent carotid bruit. It can be eliminated by carotid compression (**do not occlude carotid artery**).

Table 4.3 Evaluation of murmurs.

Technique	Details
Timing: where in the cardiac cycle they occur	If they fall between S1 and S2, they are systolic, i.e. occurring during systole (most common in children) Further, they can occur in early, mid, late or pan systole If they fall between S2 and S1, they are diastolic, i.e. occurring during diastole Further, they can occur in early, mid, late or pan diastole
Shape: the configuration that the murmur causes by its intensity over time	It can be: • crescendo: grows louder • decrescendo: grows softer • crescendo–decrescendo: grows louder and then softer • plateau: same throughout
Location of maximal intensity: the site of origin of the murmur	Can be described in terms of its relation to: • interspaces • sternum • apex • vertical lines (e.g. midclavicular)
Radiation or transmission from the point of maximal intensity: how far it radiates and where to	—
Intensity: graded 1–6	The higher the grade, the louder the murmur (Craig *et al.* 2001): (1) Very faint, difficult to hear (2) Very faint, easier to hear (3) Soft (4) Loud, associated with palpable thrill (5) Loud, can also be heard with stethoscope partially off the chest (6) Very loud, easily heard with stethoscope lifted off the chest
Pitch	Categorised as low, medium or high
Quality	Described in terms of musical, blowing or harsh

Table 4.4 Innocent and pathological murmurs.

Innocent murmurs:
- Also known as physiological, ejection or flow murmurs; are common and may be heard in up to 50% of children (Gill & O'Brien 2002)
- The following may cause innocent murmurs:
  - a closing ductus arteriosus in the newborn
  - a peripheral pulmonary flow murmur in infants
  - a venous hum (a low-pitched, continuous, rumbling murmur best heard under the right clavicle, louder when sitting up, diminishes on lying and may be abolished by obliterative pressure over the internal jugular vein; caused by blood cascading into the great veins) in early school age
- Do not increase over time
- Do not affect growth
- May disappear with change in position

Functional murmurs:
- There is no structural malformation of the heart
- There may be a physiological cause, e.g. anaemia or increased cardiac output
- The child has normal growth and development

Organic murmurs:
- A murmur is significant if it is pansystolic, conducted all over precordium, soft to loud (4–6), associated with a thrill, and accompanied by other signs, e.g. ventricular enlargement
- Children less than 3 years often have a congenital cardiac cause, e.g. valve stenosis or regurgitation
- Children over 3 years often have an acquired cardiac cause, e.g. rheumatic heart disease
- Listen over the child's back for the murmur of coarctation of the aorta
- There will be a continuous murmur in an infant with a patent ductus arteriosus (PDA) or the child who has had an arterial-pulmonary shunt (e.g. Blalock-Taussig shunt) inserted

Liver
(Advanced skill)

Estimating the size of the liver can give important information about heart failure. However, in infants, a small change in volaemic state can alter liver size (Archer & Birch 1998). Always stand on the patient's right side (Roy 1997). See Chapter 8 for technique.

Table 4.5 Common paediatric murmurs.

Name	Characteristics
Aortic stenosis Heard best with patient sitting leaning forward Use diaphragm	Mid-systolic, crescendo-decrescendo, R 2nd ICS radiating to neck/left sternal border, grade 3–4 with thrill, medium pitched, harsh
Aortic regurgitation Heard best with patient sitting up and exhaling Use diaphragm	Diastolic, decrescendo, R 2nd ICS radiating to apex if loud, grade 2–4, high pitched, blowing
Pulmonary stenosis Use diaphragm	Systolic, crescendo, L 2nd ICS, radiating to neck, grade 4, medium pitched, harsh
Mitral stenosis Use bell	Mid-diastolic, crescendo, apical, grade 1–4, low pitched, rumbling
Mitral regurgitation Use diaphragm	Pan-systolic, plateau, apical radiating to L axilla if loud, grade 3–5, medium to high pitched, blowing
Ventricular septal defect Most common CHD lesion Use diaphragm	Pan-systolic, lower L sternal border radiating over the precordium, grade 4–6, high pitched, blowing/harsh
Patent ductus arteriosus Use diaphragm	Continuous (louder in late systole), upper L sternal border, grade 2–3, medium pitched, harsh

PERIPHERAL VASCULAR ASSESSMENT
Inspection
(Basic skill)

Body posture
Check the position the child has adopted, e.g. a child with tetralogy of Fallot may squat down. This position increases peripheral resistance, thus increasing venous return and blood flow to the right side of the heart and to the lungs (increases left to right shunting of blood) (Jordan & Scott 1989).

Oedema
Look for:

- sacral, peri-orbital or flank oedema in the infant;
- oedema in the extremities of the older child.

Extremities

Observe:

- colour/symmetry/venous patterns/skin/rashes/scars;
- nailbeds for clubbing (see Chapter 2).

Palpation

(Basic skill)

Arteries

- To assess the effectiveness of circulation, it is important to palpate all arteries, including brachial, carotid and femoral, each of which have been found to be equally effective in determining a hypovolaemic state (Sarti *et al.* 2005).
- Comparison may help determine some congenital heart lesions, e.g. comparing the difference between the brachial and femoral artery may indicate coarctation of the aorta (Archer & Birch 1998).
- Pulses should be evaluated for equality, rhythm, rate and volume.

(1) *Radial and brachial arteries*: see 'Vital Signs' above.
(2) *Femoral artery*: apply deep palpation below the inguinal canal midway between anterior superior iliac spine and symphysis pubis. Infants dislike this manoeuvre and may pass urine or cry or both.
(3) *Carotid artery*: place fingers lightly on the larynx and slide laterally. This is difficult in the infant and young child due to a short neck.
(4) *Axillary artery*: place fingers in the anterior axillary line just below the head of the humerus.
(5) *Popliteal artery*: the knee is bent and the pulse detected behind the knee. The child can also be placed prone to detect the pulse. This pulse is not often examined in children.
(6) *Postero-tibialis artery*: place fingers behind and slightly below the medial malleolus of the ankle. This pulse may be difficult to detect in the chubby infant or when there is oedema.
(7) *Dorsalis pedis artery*: place fingers on the dorsum of the foot just proximal to the second toe. If you cannot feel a pulse,

explore the dorsum of the foot more laterally and change tactile sensitivity, e.g. press more lightly and then slightly harder. It can be difficult to detect this pulse in the normal chubby infant.

(8) *Pre-auricular pulse*: easily felt in the sleeping infant (Gill & O'Brien 2002).

Document
- The findings can be recorded as a descriptive paragraph or in a table. Table 4.6 shows an example.
- Note that 1+ means thready, 2+ means brisk or normal and 3+ means bounding (Bickley 2003).

Pulsus paradoxus
Pulsus paradoxus is a change in pulse volume with respiration. It is easier to detect by measuring systolic blood pressure (see 'Blood pressure' above).

Temperature of extremities
(Basic skill)
Check for warmth:

- The back of the hands are more sensitive to estimating warmth (Bickley 2003).
- Assess all the way from the tips of the extremities, moving centrally.
- Compare symmetry.

Table 4.6 Normal pulse findings.

	Carotid	Pre-auricular	Brachial	Radial	Femoral	Popliteal	Postero-tibialis	Dorsalis pedis
Left	2+	2+	2+	2+	2+	Not examined	2+	2+
Right	2+	2+	2+	2+	2+	Not examined	2+	2+

- Establish and document any coolness including the demarcation between the warmth and coolness, i.e. . . . cool to where. . . .
- Establish if the coolness is due to the environment.
- A peripheral temperature probe may be used to determine the difference between the core temperature and the peripheral temperature (suggests the volaemic state of the child – see Chapter 10).

Capillary refill
(Basic skill)

Prolonged capillary refill time (CRT) is a sign of dehydration in children (see Chapter 10). The finding is strengthened when accompanied by abnormal skin turgor and an abnormal respiratory pattern (Steiner *et al*. 2004). However, prolonged CRT must also be considered in conjunction with other clinical signs, e.g. haemodynamic instability and a rising lactate level (Cruse 2004).

Technique
- Assess one limb at a time.
- Hold limb above the level of the heart (so that gravity does not impact on the result).
- Gently squeeze a digit and hold for 5 seconds.
- Let the digit go and there should be reperfusion within 2 seconds (count . . . 1, one thousand, 2, one thousand, 3, one thousand).
- Rest the limb down.
- Document the capillary refill time as the number of seconds to reperfusion, i.e. with normal findings CRT < 2 seconds.

Normal Findings and Case Scenarios

Table 4.7 shows normal physical examination findings as well as some case studies demonstrating pathological findings for different age groups.

Table 4.7 Normal and abnormal cardiovascular findings.

INFANT
Examination techniques
Pulse – brachial, BP
Body posture
Oedema – sacral, peri-orbital, flank
Extremities – colour, skin temperature, CRT, pulses (brachial, radial, femoral, axillary, postero-tibialis, dorsalis pedis, pre-auricular)
Precordium for:

1. thrills, apical impulse
2. normal heart sounds, added heart sounds (advanced skill), murmurs (advanced skill), bruits (advanced skill)

Liver size (advanced skill)

Normal findings
Pulse 100, BP 90/60 (dynamap, right arm, 'infant'-size cuff), child supine, awake and restless
Extremities all pink, no oedema, warm, CRT < 2 sec

	Carot	Pre-aur	Brac	Rad	Fem	Pop	PT	DP
L	Not examined	2+	2+	2+	2+	Not examined	2+	2+
R	Not examined	2+	2+	2+	2+	Not examined	2+	2+

Apical impulse 4th ICS L mid-clavicular line
S1 and S2 clear, no added sounds or murmurs
No hepatomegaly

Heart failure: 6-month-old
C/V: sweating, feeding poorly
Pulse 160, BP 90/60 (dynamap, right arm, 'infant'-size cuff), child supine, awake, restless, anxious, irritable
Pale/mottled, slight peri-orbital oedema, cool peripheries, CRT 3 sec

	Carot	Pre-aur	Brac	Rad	Fem	Pop	PT	DP
L	Not examined	Not examined	1+	1+	1+	Not examined	1+	1+
R	Not examined	Not examined	1+	1+	1+	Not examined	1+	1+

Apical impulse 5th ICS L mid-clavicular line
Slight L anterior thorax bulging. Strong pulsation in infant's R xiphisternum
Gallop rhythm – no murmurs heard
Liver 4 cm below R costal margin

Continued

Table 4.7 *Continued.*

YOUNG TEENAGER
Examination techniques
Pulse – radial, BP
Body posture
Oedema – peripheral
Extremities – colour, skin temperature, CRT, clubbing, pulses (carotid, brachial, femoral, axillary, postero-tibialis, dorsalis pedis)
Precordium for:

1. bulging, heaves, lifts, thrills, apical impulse
2. normal heart sounds, added heart sounds (advanced skill), clicks (advanced skill), snaps (advanced skill), murmurs (advanced skill), bruits (advanced skill), rubs (advanced skill)

JVP (advanced skill)
Liver size (advanced skill)

Normal findings
Pulse 65, BP 110/70 (dynamap, left arm, 'small adult'-size cuff), patient sitting up and lying quietly
Extremities all pink, no oedema, no clubbing, warm, CRT <2 sec

	Carot	Pre-aur	Brac	Rad	Fem	Pop	PT	DP
L	2+	Not examined	2+	2+	2+	Not examined	2+	2+
R	2+	Not examined	2+	2+	2+	Not examined	2+	2+

Apical impulse 5th ICS L mid-clavicular line
S1 and S2 clear, no added sounds or murmurs
JVP 1 cm above sternal angle at 30°
No hepatomegaly

Hypovolaemic shock: 12-year-old
Pulse 110, BP 100/60 (dynamap, left arm, 'small adult'-size cuff), patient lying quietly
Pale and slightly mottled, no oedema, no clubbing, peripherally cool to mid-calf and wrists, CRT 4 sec

	Carot	Pre-aur	Brac	Rad	Fem	Pop	PT	DP
L	2+	Not examined	1+	1+	1+	Not examined	1+	1+
R	2+	Not examined	1+	1+	1+	Not examined	1+	1+

Apical impulse 5th ICS L mid-clavicular line
S1 and S2 clear, no added sounds or murmurs
JVP 1 cm above sternal angle at 10°
No hepatomegaly

SUMMARY

A comprehensive cardiovascular assessment can provide valuable information on the circulatory status of the patient as well as monitoring the effect of therapy. Different aspects of the examination will be useful for the health care practitioner in different clinical settings. Although the techniques of inspection, palpation and auscultation of the cardiac and vascular systems have been explored separately, it is likely that the practitioner will undertake these techniques in combination, instead focusing on less invasive approaches first prior to more invasive examination.

REFERENCES

Archer, N. & Birch, M. (1998) *Paediatric Cardiology*. Chapman and Hall Medical, London.

Bickley, L.S. (2003) *Bates Guide to Physical Examination and History Taking*, 8th edn. Lippincott, Williams and Wilkins, Philadelphia, Chapters 7, 14 and 17.

Campbell, A.G.M. & McIntosh, N. (1998) *Forfar and Arneil's Textbook of Pediatrics*, 5th edn. Churchill Livingston, New York.

Craig, J., Bloedal Smith, J. & Fineman, L.D. (2001) Tissue perfusion. In: Curley, M.A.Q. & Moloney-Harmon, P.A. (eds) *Critical Care Nursing of Infants and Children*, 2nd edn. W.B. Saunders, Philadelphia, Chapter 7.

Cruse, L. (2004) Physiological measures in intensive care. *Paediatric Nursing*, **16** (9), 14–17.

Curley, M.A.Q. & Moloney-Harmon, P.A. (2001) *Critical Care Nursing of Infants and Children*, 2nd edn. W.B. Saunders, Philadelphia.

Engel, J. (1997) *Pediatric Assessment*, 3rd edn. Mosby, St. Louis.

Gill, D. & O'Brien, N. (2002) *Paediatric Clinical Examination Made Easy*, 4th edn. Churchill Livingston, Edinburgh.

Horrox, F. (2002) *Manual of Neonatal and Paediatric Heart Disease*. Whurr, London.

Jordan, S.C. & Scott, O. (1989) *Heart Disease in Paediatrics*, 3rd edn. Butterworth Heinneman, Cambridge.

Jowett, N. (1997) *Cardiovascular Monitoring*. Whurr, London.

Park, M. & Menard, S. (1987) Accuracy of blood pressure measurements by the Dinamap monitor in infants and children. *Pediatrics*, **79** (6), 907.

Resuscitation Council (UK) (2004) *European Paediatric Life Support Course Provider Manual*. Resuscitation Council (UK), London.

Roy, D.L. (1997) Cardiovascular assessment of infants and children. In: Goldbloom, R.B. (ed) *Pediatric Clinical Skills*, 2nd edn. Churchill Livingston, Philadelphia, pp 193–217.

Sarti, A., Savron, F., Casotto, V. & Cuttini, M. (2005) Heartbeat assessment in infants: a comparison of four clinical methods. *Pediatric Critical Care Medicine*, **6** (2), 212–215.

Steiner, M.J., DeWalt, D.A. & Byerley, J.S. (2004) Is this child dehydrated? *JAMA*, **291**, 2746–2754.

Cardiovascular Monitoring and Haemodynamics

5

INTRODUCTION

Complementary to a comprehensive cardiovascular assessment is the use of electrocardiograph (ECG) and haemodynamic monitoring. ECG interpretation is essential in recognising arrhythmias that alert health care professionals to potential alteration in the patient's cardiac output.

Haemodynamics has been defined as the study of those factors that influence cardiovascular circulation (Tortora & Grabowski 2003) and include, amongst other variables, blood pressure and intracardiac pressures. Non-invasive blood pressure monitoring has been discussed within the 'Vital Signs' section of Chapter 4. The aim of this chapter is to understand the safe and accurate techniques of monitoring.

LEARNING OBJECTIVES

By the end of this chapter the reader will be able to:

❑ Appreciate the range of monitoring techniques available.
❑ Understand the effective and safe use of monitoring.
❑ Learn practical skills in using monitoring.

ELECTROCARDIOGRAPH (ECG)

As action potentials pass through the heart muscle, they produce electrical currents that can be discerned at the body surface. Therefore monitoring the ECG provides information about the electrical activity of the heart, displayed on an oscilloscope or printed out onto graph paper (Tortora & Grabowski 2003).

The calibrated graph paper that is used to record the ECG is distinctive. It has a series of heavy and light vertical and horizontal lines. Figure 5.1 shows commonly used ECG paper with a normal electrocardiogram.

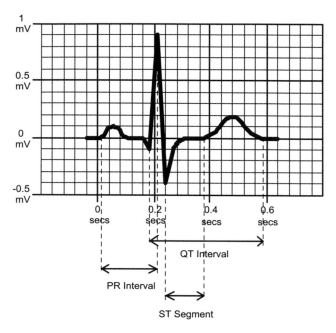

Fig. 5.1 ECG paper with a normal electrocardiogram from lead II.

The horizontal boxes measure time:

- A big square is 0.2 second and a small square is 0.04 second.
- Using this can help measure the size of the waves and intervals of the ECG complex.

The vertical lines measure voltage:

- A big square is 5 mm and is equal to 0.5 mV (millivolt); a small square is 1 mm and equals 0.1 mV.
- Using this can help determine normal and abnormal voltage size of the ECG complex.

Note that the heart is much closer to the chest wall in children and sometimes this is reflected in large complexes being recorded. It may be appropriate to repeat the recording using half sensitivity, thus making the complexes smaller and easier to interpret.

The standard speed of the ECG machine is 25 mm/second. However, it may be appropriate to stretch the ECG out in children who have fast heart rates, so that atrial activity can be more accurately evaluated. This can be achieved by using faster paper speeds of 50 or 100 mm/second.

Electrodes:

- are placed on the skin to transmit electrical impulses back to the recording machine (electrocardiograph) via the leads. Figure 5.2 shows the placement of electrodes;
- have a conductive jelly on the back that helps to decrease impedance;
- require good contact with the skin (if the body hairs cannot be moved away adequately in teenage boys, they may need to have hairs shaved);
- may require the skin being rubbed gently to remove dry skin or gently cleansed to remove slippery substances, e.g. vernix;
- may cause dermal abrasions and therefore need to be changed as per manufacturer's instructions (usually daily), although if intact, the infant may suffer dermal abrasions by the removal of electrodes;
- need to be positioned correctly to enable effective monitoring and interpretation, but for bedside monitoring the RA (right arm) and LA (left arm) electrodes may be placed on the shoulder, scapulae or top of the arms;
- come in different sizes, and smaller electrodes need to be used on infants and young children.

Leads:

- Each lead of an ECG will view the electrical activity of the heart from a different angle. Figure 5.2 shows the placement of leads.
- There are six limb leads (I, II, III, AVR, AVL, AVF) that view the heart on a frontal plane (across the chest).
- There are six chest leads (V1–V6) that view the heart in a horizontal plane (from the ribcage inwards to the heart).

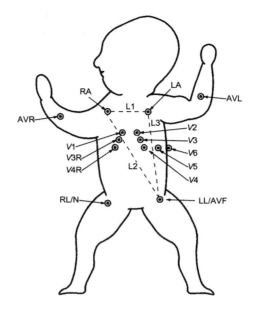

Fig. 5.2 ECG electrode placements.

By evaluating each of the leads, information can be gained on:

- the conduction pathways
- rate and rhythm
- size of the heart/chamber
- hypertrophies
- strain
- any damage in specific areas of the heart
- electrolyte levels (Craig *et al.* 2001)

Three lead ECG monitoring (standard limb leads) (leads I, II, III)
(Basic skill)

- Three lead ECG monitoring is commonly used for bedside monitoring. Figure 5.2 shows the positions of these leads.
- It is recorded as part of the 12 lead ECG.

- Two electrodes are placed above the level of the heart, one on the right side of the chest (RA) at the shoulder and one on the left (LA).
- Two electrodes are placed below the level of the heart, one on the left/centre (left leg – LL) and one on the right (right leg – RL or neutral – N).
- The neutral (N) or ground electrode could be placed anywhere but is better placed away from other leads to prevent interference. Some systems do not have the neutral electrode.

The leads are:

- bipolar (two electrodes are used as reference points; one negative and the other positive);
- labelled as RA, LA, RL/N and LL;
- attached to the electrodes;
- colour-coded for ease of use;

You may use your own 'ditty' to remember the placement of leads, e.g. 'traffic lights' – red (RA), yellow (LA), green (LL).

(Note your ditty here:)

The leads sit like cameras and detect electrical currents coming toward them (giving a positive deflection on the monitor) or going away from them (giving a negative deflection on the monitor). If the electrical current is travelling perpendicular to the 'camera' then no activity is recorded and an iso-electric baseline results (Jacobson 2000). Overall, electrical current normally flows from negative to positive:

- Lead I – detecting electrical current flowing from the negative terminal (RA) to the positive terminal (LA); normally the ECG complex should show a positive deflection on the oscilloscope.
- Lead II – detecting electrical current flowing from the negative terminal (RA) to the positive terminal (LL); normally the ECG complex should show a positive deflection on the oscilloscope.
- Lead III – detecting electrical current flowing from the negative terminal (LA) to the positive terminal (LL); normally the

ECG complex should show a positive deflection on the oscilloscope.

- Lead II most closely resembles the normal depolarisation of the heart and is therefore most commonly used for continuous monitoring (Tortora & Grabowski 2003).
- These three standard leads form a triangle known as Einthoven's triangle (Schamroth 1990).

Basic interpretation

Table 5.1 shows the basic interpretation of a bedside 3 lead ECG monitored in lead II. Figure 5.1 shows a normal electrocardiogram.

Six lead ECG (augmented unipolar limb leads) (AVR, AVL, AVF)

(Advanced skill)

- In addition to leads I, II and III, three further electrodes are placed on the child's limbs; one on each arm and one on the left leg. Figure 5.2 shows the positions of leads AVR, AVL and AVF.
- The leads are unipolar (one positive pole and a reference point). The electrodes placed on the limbs are the positive pole, the reference point being the centre of the electrical field of the heart.
- The overall electrical current detected normally flows from 'negative' or the reference point to the positive:
  - Lead AVR – detecting electrical current flowing from the 'negative' or reference point (heart) to the positive (right arm); normally the ECG complex should show a negative deflection on the oscilloscope.
  - Lead AVL – detecting electrical current flowing from the 'negative' or reference point (heart) to the positive (left arm); normally the ECG complex should show a mostly positive deflection on the oscilloscope.
  - Lead AVF – detecting electrical current flowing from the 'negative' or reference point (heart) to the positive (left foot); normally the ECG complex should show a positive deflection on the oscilloscope.

Table 5.1 Basic ECG interpretation (Schamroth 1990; Woodrow 1998; Jacobson 2000; Craig *et al.* 2001).

ECG complex	Interpretation/abnormalities
First check the child's pulse	Does it exist? (Start CPR if not) Does it match the ECG complexes on the screen? (If there is a pulse and no QRS complexes check the technical equipment and connections)
Next determine heart rate The child's age and heart rate can affect the ECG recording and intervals, e.g. there is a shorter P–R interval when the child is tachycardic. This must be taken into account alongside a table of normal values for different ages of children. See Table 4.1 for normal heart rate values	Most ECG paper has small vertical lines in the top margin at intervals, e.g. at 3- or 1-sec intervals: • for regular and irregular rhythms, count the number of R–R intervals in a 6-sec strip and multiply by 10 (to determine the rate for 1 minute); or • divide the R–R interval (count the large 5-mm boxes) into 300; or • use a rate ruler to determine heart rate Tachycardias are fast heart rates for the age of the child Bradycardias are slow heart rates for the age of the child
Then determine rhythm	Look at the graph paper to see if the rhythm is regular. A regular rhythm is called sinus rhythm Look for any irregularities, noting that a sinus arrhythmia is usually normal in children (see Chapter 4) Judge how regular the irregularity is Decide if the irregularity is fast, slow or erratic
P wave: • electrical discharge (depolarisation) from the sino-atrial (SA) node spreads across the atria, causing atrial contraction • the electrical current is travelling towards lead II and so a wave will be seen as a positive deflection on the monitor	*Ask:* Can you see P waves? Is the P wave width less than two small squares? Have the P waves a positive deflection? Do they all look the same? • a tall P wave indicates right atrial enlargement • a long P wave (may also be notched) signifies left atrial enlargement • if P waves look different they have a different origin within the atria

Continued

Table 5.1 *Continued.*

ECG complex	Interpretation/abnormalities
• when the electrical current arrives at the atrio-ventricular (AV) node, a delay is imposed, during which time atrial contraction is completed • as there is no electrical activity at this point, the monitor reflects a return to (isoelectric) baseline	

Relationship of P wave to QRS complex:
• a P wave should precede each QRS complex
P–R interval:
• this interval indicates the time from atrial depolarisation until ventricular depolarisation
	Ask:
	Is there one P wave just before every QRS complex?
	Is the P–R interval normal for the age of the child (one to two small squares in infants and two to four small squares in children)?
	A block of electrical current through the AV node can take three forms:
	(1) First degree block: there is a P wave before each QRS complex but the P–R interval is prolonged for the age of the child
	(2) Second degree block:
	  • Mobitz type I (Wenkebach): there is an increasing P–R interval until there is no P wave preceeding a QRS complex
	  • Mobitz type II: there are normal regular P waves but not all have a subsequent QRS complex
	(3) Third degree (complete heart block): there are regular P waves (faster than ventricular rate) and regular QRS complexes, but they are not at all related

QRS complex: • the electrical current emerges from the AV node and enters the Bundle of His, divides into the left and right bundle branches and then rapidly spreads throughout the purkinje fibres so that the ventricles will contract simultaneously	*Ask:* Does the QRS have a positive deflection? Is the QRS narrow? • QRS complexes are normally narrow • a widened QRS complex may indicate bundle branch block • large Q waves may indicate myocardial damage • an enlarged R wave may indicate enlarged ventricles

Table 5.1 *Continued.*

ECG complex	Interpretation/abnormalities

- the electrical current is travelling towards lead II and so a complex sharp spike will be seen as a mostly positive deflection on the monitor
- the Q wave depicts depolarisation of the ventricular septum and is a small negative wave
- the R wave depicts left ventricular activity and is the first positive deflection
- the S wave depicts right ventricular activity and is a negative deflection following an R wave
- if a complex is all positive, it is called an R wave
- if a complex is all negative, it is called a QS wave
- the height of the R and S waves reflects the thickness of the ventricular wall

Q–T interval:
- this interval indicates the time from ventricular depolarisation to ventricular repolarisation

Increases with slower heart rates and vice versa.

Ask:

Is it bigger than two big squares?

Are there any changes from the previous ECG?

A prolonged Q–T interval may indicate:
- hypocalcaemia
- hypokalaemia
- hypomagnesaemia
- myocarditis
- conduction abnormalities, e.g. bundle branch block
- drugs, e.g. amiodorone, procainamide
- long QT syndrome

A shortened Q–T interval may indicate:
- hypercalcaemia
- hyperkalaemia
- a patient on digoxin therapy

Continued

Table 5.1 *Continued.*

ECG complex	Interpretation/abnormalities
S–T segment: • this interval indicates the time between the end of depolarisation and the beginning of repolarisation • as there is no electrical activity at this point, the monitor reflects a return to (isoelectric) baseline	*Ask:* Does the trace return to the isoelectric baseline between S and T? A raised interval suggests: • myocardial infarction • pericarditis A depressed segment indicates: • myocardial ischaemia • digoxin therapy
T wave: • the ventricles relax as re-polarisation occurs • the electrical current is travelling towards lead II and so a wave will be seen as a mostly positive deflection on the monitor • the T waves are smaller and wider than the QRS complex because repolarisation occurs more slowly than depolarisation	*Ask:* Does the T wave have a positive deflection? T waves that are taller than normal indicate: • hyperkalaemia (with increasing K+ levels, the QRS complex then also widens) • myocardial ischaemic changes Inverted T waves can be caused by: • ischaemia • infarction • myocarditis Flat T waves can be seen in: • hypothyroidism • hypokalaemia • myocarditis • pericardial effusion, accompanied by small voltage QRS complexes

Combining Einthoven's triangle of the standard leads with the limb leads in a diagrammatic fashion gives a reference system known as the frontal plane hexaxial reference system. This system allows practitioners to determine the electrical axis of the heart and accurate evaluation of abnormalities such as myocardial infarction, bundle branch block and hypertrophies (Schamroth 1990). This is not discussed further in this book.

Twelve lead ECG
(Advanced skill)
When undertaking a 12 lead ECG, there are only 10 leads as some leads within this procedure have a dual role. A lead is

placed on each limb and six further electrodes are placed across the patient's chest. Figure 5.2 shows the positions of these chest leads V1–V6.

The chest electrodes and leads are placed in specific intercostals spaces (ICS): walk your fingers down the rib cage from the clavicle to determine correct positioning:

- V1 – 4th RICS (right intercostal space) adjacent to sternum; detecting electrical current flowing from the 'negative' or reference point (heart) to the positive (V1); normally the ECG complex should show a negative deflection on the oscilloscope.
- V2 – 4th LICS (left intercostal space) adjacent to sternum; detecting electrical current flowing from the 'negative' or reference point (heart) to the positive (V2); normally the ECG complex should show a negative deflection on the oscilloscope.
- V4 – 5th LICS midclavicular line; detecting electrical current flowing from the 'negative' or reference point (heart) to the positive (V4); normally the ECG complex should show a balanced positive and negative deflection on the oscilloscope.
- V3 – midway between V2 and V4; detecting electrical current flowing from the 'negative' or reference point (heart) to the positive (V3); normally the ECG complex should show a balanced but slightly more negative deflection on the oscilloscope.
- V5 – 5th LICS anterior axilla line; detecting electrical current flowing from the 'negative' or reference point (heart) to the positive (V5); normally the ECG complex should show a positive deflection on the oscilloscope.
- V6 – 5th LICS mid-axilla line; detecting electrical current flowing from the 'negative' or reference point (heart) to the positive (V6); normally the ECG complex should show a positive deflection on the oscilloscope.

Groups of the 12 lead ECG look at specific areas of the heart (Schamroth 1990):

- inferior surface of the heart – II, III, AVF
- superior left lateral wall – I, AVL

- cavity of heart – AVR, V1
- anterior left ventricle – AVL, V4–V6
- anterior right ventricle – V1, V2
- posterior heart – nil

Right-side chest leads

(Advanced skill)

The 12 lead ECG recording in infants and young children can include V3R or V4R or both (Archer & Birch 1998). These leads are placed on the right side of the chest in the same positions as those corresponding on the left (see Fig. 5.2 for placement positions):

- In infancy, there is a right ventricular dominancy and axis and this recording helps to evaluate the right heart.
- In infancy, the normal positive and negative deflections in V1–V6 leads are changed due to this right ventricular dominancy.
- In childhood these leads may determine right ventricular enlargement.

Trouble-shooting

- Minimise the number of electrical appliances at the bedside to prevent electrical interference/artefact (artefact meaning anything on the ECG that is not of cardiac origin).
- Keep the child warm and calm to prevent muscle tremor.
- Ensure good skin contact with electrodes correctly placed.
- Normal breathing should prevent a wandering baseline.

CARDIAC INDEX

Absolute blood volumes are small in infants (80 ml/kg); however, in relation to their body weight, infants and children have greater cardiac outputs than adults. Normal cardiac outputs (COs) are:

- Infant: 200 ml/kg/min
- Child: 150 ml/kg/min
- Young person: 100 ml/kg/min (Horrox 2002)

For practical purposes, the cardiac index (CI) is a more useful tool to evaluate cardiac output (Webster 1992). CI normal is 2.5–5 L/min/m² (Craig *et al.* 2001).

First the body surface area (BSA), measured in square metres (m²), needs calculating:

$$BSA \ (m^2) = \frac{height \ (cm) \times weight \ (kg)}{3600}$$

Then

$$CI = \frac{CO \ (litres)}{BSA \ (m^2)}$$

For example: a 10-year-old child is 30 kg in weight and 1.35 m tall:

$$BSA = \frac{135 \ (cm) \times 30 \ (kg)}{3600} = 1.125$$

$$CI = \frac{150 \times 30/1000 \ (CO, \ in \ litres)}{1.125 \ (BSA)} = 4 \ L/min/m^2$$

A simple internet search will provide automated calculations for you.

TRANSDUCERS

Transducers are used within critical care areas, where normal body physiological control mechanisms are severely damaged. They transform one type of energy to another, e.g. they detect the mechanical pressure waves of the vascular system/organ tissue and change them to an electrical signal that is sent to a monitor and displayed on an oscilloscope (Webster 1992).

Transducers are attached to a catheter to acquire this physiological information. Cardiac pressures as well as brain tissue amongst other body structures can be monitored in this way. Use of transducers requires specific training of health care professionals. Figure 5.3 shows a transducer system attached to a radial arterial line.

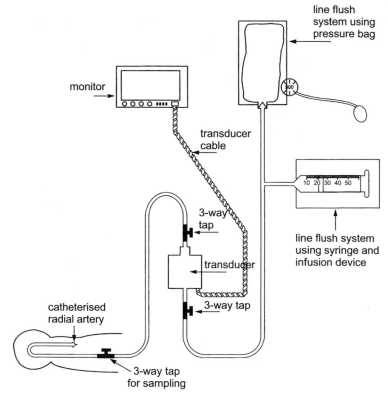

Fig. 5.3 A transducer attached to a radial arterial line.

Requirements

A transducer system requires:

(1) *A monitor*
These usually self-calibrate.

(2) *A transducer*
Most transducers are now disposable, do not need calibrating and use a microchip for sensing.

(3) *A flush system*

Where the cardiovascular system is being monitored, flushing the line prevents emboli occlusion of the vascular catheter and back-flow of blood into the transducer. Exceptions may include:

- a left atrial monitoring line (depending on local protocol) where there may be a risk of air getting into the left side of the heart;

(*Note your clinical area's policy here:*)

- a central venous line where the central catheter is being used as a fluid or drug line. Large volumes may be administered, hence a flushing system is not required to maintain catheter patency. However, the fluid or drug infusion may have to be turned off momentarily to achieve an accurate CVP reading.

The flushing fluid (when used) is usually normal saline and may have heparin added. Although evidence for the use of heparin is unclear, there appears to be an argument for the addition of heparin in infants and young children (Butt *et al.* 1987; Rogier *et al.* 2005).

(*Note your clinical area's policy here:*)

The flush is normally delivered via an infusion pump (especially in infants and small children) or a high-pressure bag, although these are much less accurate (Metz & Whitford 1996).

(*Note your clinical area's policy here:*)

Continuous flushing is less likely to distort the pressure waves on the oscilloscope and increases longevity of catheter patency.

(4) *Ports for access*

A port at the transducer sensor allows 'zeroing' of the transducer (see below). A port at the catheter site facilitates any requirement for sampling. When using an heparinised flush system a larger dead space of blood must be drawn when sampling blood for coagulation profiles. When aspirating the catheter for blood sampling, check that:

- universal precautions and a clean, non-touch technique are used;
- the three-way tap (access point) near the catheter insertion site has its cap removed and discarded;
- this access point is cleaned with alcohol and allowed to dry;
- the syringe is then attached to the clean access point;
- then the three-way tap is turned off to the flush and on to the patient, so the syringe can aspirate a 1- to 2-ml deadspace sample (taken prior to the true sample);
- once aspiration is complete, the three-way tap is turned diagonally so that it is off to the access point and the patient;
- the deadspace sample is removed and placed on a clean surface (often placed back in the syringe packet) and a new syringe is used to aspirate the true sample(s);
- once aspiration is complete, the three-way tap is turned diagonally so that it is off to the access point and the patient;
- the true sample is removed and the deadspace blood is returned to the child to prevent iatrogenic hypovolemia and anaemia (particularly in the infant and young child). Note that there is some evidence to suggest that microbubbles and fibrin platelet aggregate may be pushed into the arterial system and to the brain (Butt *et al.* 1985). Inject this sample very slowly to reduce the risk of arterial spasm;
- the deadspace syringe is removed and a fresh syringe with 1–2 ml of normal saline is used to gently flush the line (not the continuous flow infusion as it is unknown how much is being administered) (Webster 1992);
- the access point is cleaned with alcohol and allowed to dry before placing a new cap;
- the child's limb is assessed for good perfusion (warmth, pulses, CRT) and the arterial waveform on the monitor is examined for a normal contour.

(5) *Low compliance tubing*

Mechanical energy can be absorbed into compliant tubing, giving dampened and inaccurate waveforms. Clear short tubing allows for continual observation for air bubbles and clots and the minimal amount of journey for the pressure wave.

(6) *A one-way valve*

To allow small volumes (1–3 ml) of flushing fluid through the transducer on a continuous basis and to prevent backflow.

Continuous assessment

A transducer system needs continuous assessment to maintain adequate waveforms. Check:

- all connections of the transducer and lines are intact, and with tight connections;
- all three-way taps are turned so that there is no backflow of patient blood;
- there is no air (often accumulates in three-way taps or near the sensor), clots, bubbles or kinking in the lines (flush any air or clots through the system with the three-way tap turned off to the patient);
- there is adequate continuous flushing of fluid through the line (according to local protocol) to prevent thrombi formation:
  - o the infusion pump is running at the prescribed rate (1–3 ml/hour);
  - o the pressure bag pressure is kept at 300 mmHg for approximately 3 ml/hour and 200 mmHg for approximately 2 ml/hour;
  - o the flushing device must run at a volume that will overcome the child's own blood pressure, to prevent bleedback (Webster 1992);
- an appropriate scale on the oscilloscope is being used with individual waveforms to ensure appropriate waveforms, e.g. if the arterial pressure is 90/50 then the scale must be higher than 90 and lower than 50.

Zeroing

The transducer is zeroed when first set up and whenever the lead is disconnected from the monitor. It may be local protocol to zero on a more regular basis.

(*Note your clinical area's policy here:*)

Zeroing means that a reference point of zero is used to measure haemodynamics. Normal atmospheric pressure is 760 mmHg at sea level. Opening the transducer to air and making the monitor read atmospheric pressure as zero allows the haemodynamic monitoring values to be isolated from the impact of atmospheric pressure.

When intracardiac pressures are being monitored, the transducer is levelled at the right atrium. This phlebostatic axis can be at the:

- 4th intercostal space mid-axilla line; or
- 4th intercostal space at the sternum (*tick which one you use in your unit*).

When patients are moved, their phlebostatic axis reference point needs to be checked. It is important to be as accurate as possible in monitoring haemodynamics, particularly if the results mean the institution or manipulation of fluid, drug or technical therapies.

A spirit level piece (or a piece of flexible tubing connected to make a circle and half-filled with coloured fluid) is used for accuracy in ensuring the transducer is at the right phlebostatic axis point. Zeroing should follow manufacturer's instructions but is commonly undertaken as follows:

(1) Turn the three-way tap at the transducer level so that it is 'off' to the patient and 'on' so that the transducer will be exposed to air once the cap is removed. This will automatically mean that the flush is off (but see below*).

(2) Remove the cap to the three-way tap at the transducer level.

(3) Press the 'zero' button on the monitor and wait for the value to settle on 0.

(4) Replace the three-way tap cap.

(5) Turn the three-way tap at the transducer back to the position where it is 'off' to the air and 'on' to the patient.
(6) This will automatically mean the flush will now run.

*If you have pressed stop on the flush you may need to press start again.

When more than one haemodynamic parameter is being measured, all transducers should be placed in the same holder to be able to compare information. Abnormal readings must be correlated with a clinical examination and be a cue to check the phlebostatic level of the transducer and the zeroing.

HAEMODYNAMIC MONITORING

Transducers are attached to vascular catheters for haemodynamic monitoring. Vascular cannulation of arteries, large veins and intracardiac chambers can be used (see below for discussion of each). Careful consideration must be given to setting alarm limits: ask 'At what point do I want to know that parameter has changed?'. Table 5.2 shows the uses and general complications of haemodynamic monitoring (Craig *et al.* 2001).

Requirements

Catheters need continual assessment:

- It is useful for the site to be visible at all times.
- Maintain an intact dressing.
- Monitor the catheter site for bleeding, inflammation or infection.

Table 5.2 Haemodynamic monitoring.

Can give information on:	Has potential complications including:
• preload and afterload	• infection
• right and left heart function	• haemorrhage
• vascular resistances	• embolus
• intracardiac shunting	• pneumothorax
• valve competency	• arrhythmias
• response to fluid, drug (inotropes or vasodilators) or technical therapies (pacing)	• malpositioning
	• cardiac tamponade
	• ischaemic limbs

- Ensure the cannula and line are well secured, to prevent dislodgement as well as lodgement against the vessel wall (when this occurs, reposition patient or restrap catheter).
- Ensure the cannula and line are well labelled; there should be no ambiguity about appropriate vascular access during the normal course of fluid and drug administration or in an emergency situation.
- Ensure the limb is kept in alignment to prevent kinking of the cannula, e.g. the hand and forearm of a child who has a radial cannula may have the hand positioned and strapped supine on a splint.
- Monitor the distal limb for circulation including pulses, warmth and capillary refill time.

ARTERIAL CATHETERS AND INTRA-ARTERIAL BLOOD PRESSURE (IABP) MONITORING
Arterial catheters
Arterial lines are used within critical care areas and specific training is required prior to use. An arterial line is inserted for two reasons:

- blood gas analysis (see Chapter 3);
- invasive, continuous blood pressure monitoring.

Any arteries can be used for monitoring blood pressure but most commonly the radial (do not use the left radial artery in infants with coarctation of the aorta), femoral, brachial (can decrease perfusion to arm), axilla, dorsalis pedis and umbilical arteries in newborns are used.

Arteries exert higher pressures than veins and therefore puncturing of arteries can produce significant bleeding. It is thus vital that an arterial catheter and line is always able to be seen. Drugs or drug infusions are not routinely administered through an arterial line. It is vital that an arterial line is extremely well labelled with very clear identification.

(*Note your clinical area's policy here:*)

Intra-arterial blood pressure monitoring
The arterial waveform should demonstrate the anacrotic notch, the peak systolic pressure reflecting left ventricular systolic

pressure. Also the dicrotic notch; the aortic valve closing causes a small increase in pressure in the artery (may be decreased in low cardiac output states) and the diastolic pressure, reflecting the vasoconstriction in the arterial system. The dicrotic notch may not be seen in arteries other than the radial and axilla arteries (Civetta *et al*. 1997). Normal blood pressure values apply (see Table 4.2 for normal values). Figure 5.4 shows a normal waveform.

Pulse pressure is the difference between the systolic and diastolic values. It gives information on the stroke volume and ability for the stroke volume to be delivered into the arterial system. Table 5.3 shows some causes of pulse pressure abnormalities.

A flat line on the monitor may indicate that the artery has gone into spasm (excluding cardiac collapse):

- Rest the limb and allow time for the spasm to pass.
- It may be helpful to apply warmth to the opposite limb to try to induce vasodilation.

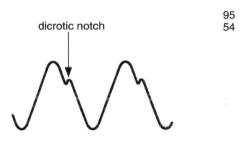

Fig. 5.4 Normal arterial waveform.

Table 5.3 Pulse pressure abnormalities.

Narrow pulse pressure	Wide pulse pressure
Causes:	Causes:
• hypovolaemia	• Blalock-Taussig shunt
• increased systemic vascular resistance	

- Check that the flush is on, but giving extra flush is often not helpful.
- Forceful flushing should not be attempted.

A dampened trace may require the cannula to be aspirated carefully using short, quick 'pulls' to loosen and retrieve the clot and then flushed with a small amount of normal saline. Forceful flushing should not be attempted.

Some local policies may request that the intra-arterial blood pressure values are 'checked' against a manual blood pressure. In normal patients, the direct measurement of mechanical pulse pressures through invasive monitoring may be similar to the measurement of Karotkoff's sounds of auscultation or the oscillations of pulsatile blood flow returning to a compressed artery, but this may not be the case with a child who is critically ill. There is poor correlation between different methods (Park & Menard 1987). The problem becomes which to believe and, more importantly, which to treat?

Manipulation and handling of the catheter
- Handle the catheter, tubing and three-way taps minimally.
- Any blanching of the skin that occurs with flushing needs consideration of catheter replacement.
- Any blanching that does not subside means immediate removal of the catheter.
- The catheter should not be opened to the air; manipulation of the three-way tap and syringes can be undertaken to prevent this.
- Use universal precautions, effective hand cleaning techniques and gloves.
- Change the tubing and three-way taps as per local policy (usually every 3–4 days using a clean, non-touch technique).

(*Note your clinical area's policy here:*)

Removal of catheter
Once continuous blood pressure monitoring (and blood gas analysis) is no longer required, the catheter should be removed as soon as possible. Check that:

- dressings are removed;
- any sutures that may have been placed are removed;
- any blood is cleaned away from the catheter site with gauze and sterile water;
- a clean piece of gauze is used to place some pressure on the catheter entry site;
- the other hand is used to withdraw the catheter continuously, maintaining pressure on the site;
- the catheter is examined, ensuring it is complete;
- pressure is maintained on the site for at least 5 minutes, longer if the patient's clotting profile is prolonged;
- a small dressing can be applied once all oozing has stopped and there is no evidence of a haematoma forming;
- pressure dressings are not recommended;
- the site is frequently observed after removal, checking for oozing and haematoma formation;
- the dressing is removed after 24 hours if the wound is clean.

CENTRAL LINES AND CENTRAL VENOUS PRESSURE (CVP) MONITORING

This type of monitoring is seen in the very sick child and specific training in managing these lines is required.

Long-term catheters

These are not considered in detail here. They are:

- usually tunnelled or implanted (port);
- used in oncology or with children requiring long-term parenteral nutrition.

Short-term catheters

These are usually percutaneously inserted and used in acute illness, e.g. in the intensive care or high-dependency unit. Large volumes of fluid and drugs/infusions (sometimes in higher concentrations) can be administered. Insertion may be central (jugular, femoral, subclavian) or peripheral (cubital, saphenous in newborns) (de Jonge et al. 2005). The central catheter can be used for blood sampling. However, due to the low pressure in the right atrium and the fall of the pressure on expiration, care needs to be taken with opening the three-way tap. The pressure outside the catheter, particularly if the three-way tap is raised above the level of the heart, may be enough to cause air to be be sucked into the catheter and right atrium, so it is important to manipulate the three-way tap so that at no time is the internal diameter of the catheter exposed to the air.

The catheter should be well secured as displacement is easy in a restless, very young or inquisitive child (de Jonge *et al.* 2005). An X-ray is recommended following insertion:

- to check correct position;
- to look for complications such as pnemothorax (with subclavian or jugular vein access) (de Jonge *et al.* 2005).

Look for thrombus formation (occurs at the tip or at the site where the catheter penetrates the vessel wall), especially in the small child who has had a catheter in situ for a while:

- Aspirate a little blood with a syringe prior to administering fluids or drugs and judge how easy the aspiration is.
- Observe for any swelling or oedema at the catheter site, where the tip of the catheter would be and beyond; it is often localised to the arm, neck and face of the affected side (de Jonge *et al.* 2005).

Superior vena cava syndrome can occur with catheters positioned in the superior vena cava (Craig *et al.* 2001). Thrombus formation in this area can obstruct venous return from the head. The head and neck become swollen and discoloured. Drug therapy (fibrinolytics) or surgical intervention may be required to remove the clot.

As per local protocol, flush the line intermittently or continuously. Normal saline, heparin (no strong evidence) or urokinase may be used (de Jonge *et al.* 2005).

Infection

Colonisation and bacteraemia infection are a significant risk (de Jonge *et al.* 2005) and there is an increased risk with:

- parenteral nutrition;
- a percutaneously inserted catheter;
- multiple lumens;

- more frequent manipulation and handling of the catheter (keep handling to a minimum);
- increased severity of illness;
- lack of evidence-based protocols and staff education (Puntis *et al.* 1991; Lange *et al.* 1997);
- high risk of contamination, e.g. blood, saliva, secretions, critical illness (use universal precautions, effective hand cleaning techniques and gloves).

Changing the infusion lines and three-way taps every 72 hours (blood product and lipid sets every 24 hours) in an aseptic/clean technique (as per local policy) reduces infection risk.

(*Note your clinical area's policy here:*)

The use of in-line filters may reduce the risk, but this has not been well demonstrated (de Jonge *et al.* 2005). The child needs to be assessed for clinical signs of infection (fever, cold chills, malaise, haemodynamic instability, raised WCC (white cell count) and CRP).

Central venous pressure (CVP) monitoring
(Advanced skill)

CVP reflects the right atrial pressure and monitoring assists with decision-making in fluid administration. It is useful to have the tip of the catheter at the cavo-atrial junction (confirmed on chest X-ray). The waveform shape reflects the normally low pressure found in the right atrium and has an A wave reflecting right atrial contraction, a C wave formed by the tricuspid valve closure and a V wave which reflects the pressure from ventricular contraction. The waveform rises with spontaneous inspiration and falls on expiration (Kaussmaul waves). Table 5.4 shows a normal waveform.

Measuring the CVP gives information on the right atrial pressure reflecting:

- the patient's blood volume (preload);
- right ventricular function (if the right ventricle is in failure, the pressure may reflect back into the right atrium, raising the CVP);
- indirectly the pulmonary vascular system pressures.

Table 5.4 Right atrial pressure – normal and abnormal findings.

Right atrial pressure waveform and values	Causes of abnormal pressures
Normal waveform Normal pressures 0–6 mmHg	Possible causes of high pressure: • cardiac tamponade • heart failure • fluid overload Possible causes of low pressure: • hypovolaemia • reduced pulmonary venous return

The CVP measures pressure within the right atrium and therefore any other cause of increased intrathoracic pressure will be reflected in the CVP, e.g. positive pressure ventilation will increase the CVP as well as obliterating the Kaussmaul waves (may get a flatter wave).

Removal of central catheter

- The child lies down as flat as possible to reduce the risk of air entering the catheter during removal.
- Removal on end-inspiration may be helpful, when intrathoracic pressure is highest and decreases the risk of air entering the catheter (Craig *et al.* 2001).
- Using universal precautions, the dressing is removed.
- Any sutures that may have been placed are removed.
- Any blood is cleaned away from the catheter site with gauze and sterile water.
- A clean piece of gauze is used to place some pressure on the catheter entry site.
- The other hand is used to withdraw the catheter continuously, maintaining pressure on the site.
- ECG monitoring in situ can be helpful to check for arrhythmias during removal.
- The catheter is examined, ensuring its complete removal.
- The tip may be sent for culture if indicated.
- Pressure is maintained on the site for at least 3 minutes, longer if the patient's clotting profile is prolonged.

- Once all oozing has stopped and there is no evidence of a haematoma forming, a small dressing can be applied.
- Pressure dressings are not recommended.
- The site should be frequently observed after catheter removal, checking for oozing.
- The dressing is removed after 24 hours if the wound is clean.

INTRACARDIAC HAEMODYNAMIC MONITORING

Catheters can be placed directly into the chambers of the heart and pulmonary artery and brought out through the skin at the time of cardiac surgery. This type of monitoring is used when clinical decision-making would benefit from having this information. The presence of these lines provides a significant risk to the child and must be managed following specific training. The catheters are attached to transducers to monitor the waveforms and values.

Intracardiac left atrial pressure (LAP)

A direct catheter into the left atrium of the heart will give information on:

- atrial filling pressure;
- left ventricular end-diastole filling pressure. Table 5.5 shows normal waveforms and pressures and causes of abnormal findings.

Table 5.5 Left atrial pressure – normal and abnormal findings.

Left atrial pressure waveform and values	Causes of abnormal pressures
Normal waveform Normal pressures 2–10 mmHg	Possible causes of high pressure: • cardiac tamponade • fluid overload Possible causes of low pressure: • hypovolaemia • reduced pulmonary venous return

Specific points of care (Craig *et al.* 2001)
- No drugs are normally administered.
- Depending on local policy, the line may or may not have a continuous flushing infusion.
- Observe closely for air or clots in the line or catheter; if any are found the three-way tap must be turned off immediately.
- Clots and air may be aspirated, but manual flushing must be undertaken with medical orders.
- Any blood aspirated must not be returned to the patient to prevent the risk of air or a clot being injected.
- Monitor the neurological status of the patient (see Chapter 7).
- Monitor ECG and observe for arrhythmias.
- Observe for signs of cardiac tamponade from bleeding into the pericardial space.

Intracardiac right atrial pressure
A direct catheter into the right atrium of the heart will give the same information as the central venous pressure discussed above.

Intracardiac pulmonary artery pressure
A direct catheter into the pulmonary artery of the heart will provide information on the systolic, mean and diastolic pulmonary artery pressures and the effectiveness of the right ventricular function as well as the stability of the pulmonary vasculature. These haemodynamic parameters can assist in decision-making concerning the instigation of appropriate fluid, drug and mechanical therapy or its manipulation.

The pulmonary artery catheter is not used routinely for administration of drugs. However, pulmonary dilators may be prescribed to be administered via this route. Blood can be sampled for interpretation of mixed venous gases.

Early recognition of an impending pulmonary hypertensive crisis can help with early management (this can occur following cardiac surgery for repair of large left to right lesions, e.g. atrioventricular septal defect). Table 5.6 shows causes of high pulmonary artery pressures.

Table 5.6 Normal and abnormal pulmonary artery pressures.

Pulmonary artery pressure waveform and values	Causes of high pressures
Normal waveform Normal pressures (one-third of systemic pressure): Systolic: 20–30 Mean: 7–18 Diastolic: 4–12	• Increased pulmonary blood flow (from left to right shunting) • Increased resistance to pulmonary blood flow (e.g. pulmonary disease, pulmonary hypertension, pulmonary embolus or severe heart failure)

Removal of intracardiac haemodynamic monitoring catheters

Check:

- the local policy for:
  - patient clotting/coagulation status requirements;
  - blood availability requirements;
  - personnel permitted to perform this procedure;
  - personnel to be informed of the procedure, e.g. surgeon;
- timing of the catheter removal, which is locally determined but may be either:
  - prior to the removal of chest drains so that any bleeding into the chest can be drained; or
  - after 5–7 days of having been 'tied off' (catheters are disconnected from transducers and flushing systems and then capped or tied);
- using universal precautions, the dressing is removed;
- any sutures that may have been placed are removed;
- any blood is cleaned away from the catheter site with gauze and sterile water;
- that a clean piece of gauze is used to cover the catheter entry site;
- the other hand is used to withdraw the catheter continuously;

- there may be a sense of pulling a little firmly and then a sudden slight 'give';
- ECG monitoring in situ is useful to check for arrhythmias during removal;
- the catheter is examined ensuring its complete removal;
- pressure is maintained on the site for a couple of minutes, longer if the patient's clotting profile is prolonged;
- that once all oozing has stopped and there is no evidence of a haematoma forming, a small dressing can be applied;
- pressure dressings are not recommended;
- the site is observed frequently after removal, checking for oozing;
- that an echocardiogram is booked to check for bleeding post-removal if part of the local policy;
- the dressing is removed after 24 hours if wound is clean.

The health care practitioner must be vigilant for signs of cardiac tamponade (bleeding around the heart causing compression of the ventricles and decreased cardiac output). Look for and report as a medical emergency:

- neck vein distension
- hypotension
- narrow pulse pressure
- widened mediastinum on chest X-ray

SUMMARY

ECG and haemodynamic monitoring are used as part of the care to some degree of all children who are unwell. Clinicians need to decide on the level of monitoring required to assist with clinical decision-making on the use of and response to drugs, fluids and therapies. All technology requires accurate and safe use by the health care professional as well as for the patient.

REFERENCES

Archer, N. & Birch, M. (1998) *Paediatric Cardiology*. Chapman and Hall Medical, London.

Butt, W., Gow, R., Whyte, H., Smallhorn, J. & Koren, G. (1985) Complications resulting from use of arterial catheters, retrograde flow and rapid elevation in blood pressure. *Paediatrics*, **76** (2), 250–253.

Butt, W., Shann, F., McDonnell, G. & Hudson, I. (1987) Effect of heparin concentration and infusion rate on the patency of arterial catheters. *Critical Care Medicine*, **15** (3), 230–232.

Civetta, R.W., Taylor, R.W. & Kirby, R.R. (1997) *Critical Care*. Lippincott, Philadelphia.

Craig, J., Bloedal Smith, J. & Fineman, L.D. (2001) Tissue perfusion. In: Curley, M.A.Q. & Moloney-Harmon, P.A. (eds) *Critical Care Nursing of Infants and Children*, 2nd edn. W.B. Saunders, Philadelphia, Chapter 7.

de Jonge, R.C.J., Polderman, K.H. & Gemke, R.J.B.J. (2005) Central venous catheter use in the pediatric patient: mechanical and infectious complications. *Pediatric Critical Care Medicine*, **6** (3), 329–339.

Horrox, F. (2002) *Manual of Neonatal and Paediatric Heart Disease*. Whurr, London.

Jacobson, S. (2000) Electrocardiography. In: Woods, S.L., Froelicher, E.S.S. & Motzer, S.U. (eds) *Cardiac Nursing*. Lippincott, Philadelphia.

Lange, B.J., Weiman, M. & Feuer, E.J. (1997) Impact of changes in catheter management on infectious complications among children with central venous catheters. *Infectious Control Hospital Epidemiology*, **18**, 326–332.

Metz, L.C. & Whitford, K. (1996) Fluid delivery by pressure monitoring systems in the pediatric intensive care unit: a retrospective comparative analysis of two systems. *American Journal of Critical Care*, **5** (1), 66–67.

Park, M. & Menard, S. (1987) Accuracy of blood pressure measurements by the Dinamap monitor in infants and children. *Pediatrics*, **79** (6), 907.

Puntis, J.W., Holden, C.E. & Smallman, S. (1991) Staff training: a key factor in reducing intravascular catheter sepsis. *Archives of Disease in Childhood*, **66**, 335–337.

Schamroth, C. (ed) (1990) *An Introduction to Electrocardiography*, 7 edn. Blackwell, Oxford.

Tortora, G.J. & Grabowski, S.R. (2003) *Principles of Anatomy and Physiology*, 10th edn. John Wiley, New York.

Webster H. (1992) Bioinstrumentation: principles and techniques. In: Hazinski, M.F. (ed) *Nursing Care of the Critically Ill Child*, 2nd edn. Mosby, St Louis, Chapter 14.

Woodrow, P. (1998) An introduction to the reading of electrocardiograms. *British Journal of Nursing*, **7** (13), 135–142.

6 | Neurological Assessment

INTRODUCTION

Due to the nature of the immaturity of the neurological system and development within different age groups, neurological assessment is challenging. Getting co-operation from the child is essential and the examiner needs to use effective strategies to gain this co-operation. Neurological abnormalities often present as developmental abnormalities and so these examinations go hand-in-hand. Regression may occur when the child is hospitalised, compounded by separation from family and normal home routine and as a consequence of the illness. Mental health is not discussed in this book. The overall aim of this chapter is to understand the rationale for assessment and to undertake accurate techniques.

LEARNING OBJECTIVES

By the end of this chapter the reader will be able to:

❏ Understand and use normal developmental stages to evaluate neurological function in different age groups.
❏ Consider aspects of history as an important part of neurological examination.
❏ Undertake neurological physical assessment in different age groups.

NORMAL GROWTH AND DEVELOPMENT

(see Tables 6.1–6.8)
(Basic skill)
Although this book focuses on assessment and monitoring of the sick child, it is pertinent to understand normal growth and

Table 6.1 Normal growth and development of the neonate.

Posture and gross motor movements	Vision and fine motor movements
• Hypertonic arms and legs and hypotonic neck and trunk • Held prone (hold with both hands around the trunk), the head drops forward and arms and legs are flexed • Held in a sitting position (grasp both infant's hands and pull to sitting position), the head lags and then falls forward • Lying supine, the baby's arms and legs are flexed • Arms more so than legs begin to have jerky movements at about 1 month • The head turns to one side at 1 month	• See primitive reflexes below • Turn baby's head towards a significant source of light • No accommodation, so objects must be within 30 cm for baby to fix on it • Will follow a face if turned slowly, and by 1 month will focus and watch a familiar nearby face • Pupils react to light by 1 month • Bright or bold toys will hold attention if in close proximity (20–30 cm) • Will have blink at 6–8 weeks

Hearing and speech	Social behaviour and play
• See primitive reflexes below • Cannot localise sound but will cease movement temporarily when a noise is elicited, e.g. bell, by 1 month • By 1 month will stop any minor grizzling to turn towards a noise but not if screaming or feeding • Will cry loudly by 1 month if uncomfortable or hungry	• Sleeps most of the time • Has eye contact with carer • Exhibits facial gestures towards carer • Becoming more alert by 4–6 weeks, with smiles and responsive babbling • By 1 month will grasp objects if put into palm

development so that appropriate approaches are used and findings are contextual. Where there is developmental delay or special needs of children, the profile of development will be different from the majority of children but normal for the affected child.

Although there is a wide variation of normal growth and development, any concerns by the family or health care

Table 6.2 Normal growth and development of the infant at 3–6 months.

Posture and gross motor movements	Vision and fine motor movements
• Head stays in midline when lying supine • Limbs are less jerky, kicking more vigorously, and by 6 months infant is grasping feet • Head has less lag, back is straighter and by 6 months infant has a straight back with erect head, is sitting with support and looking around • Lifts head when lying prone and by 6 months infants are supporting themselves with their arms extended • Knees buckle when infant stood up but become weight-bearing by 6 months	• Much more alert and watching nearby objects and faces; will move head to follow • Watches own hands; places palms of hands together; plays with fingers • Eyes will converge if object moved towards face • May hold a rattle for a few seconds and wave it • By 6 months purposefully follows activities in the room • Eyes move together and a squint is abnormal at 6 months • Stretches both hands to grasp objects at 6 months • At 6 months passes objects from one hand to the other with a palmar grasp • Outwith visual field, a dropped object is only briefly looked for when 6 months old

Hearing and speech	Social behaviour and play
• Sudden and loud noises are still distressing • May look as if searching for a noise by moving head side to side, but by 6 months will turn directly to the source of noise if very close by • Will become quiet and smiles with familiar voice or toy noises except when very distressed • Will babble with pleasure and by 6 months laugh • Will become excited at the sound of familiar noises, e.g. footsteps, bath water running • By 6 months will listen to someone's voice even if cannot see anyone • Appears to be 'singing' to self by 6 months with single sounds, e.g. 'goo' • Can squeal with pleasure and cry out loudly with displeasure by 6 months	• Gazes at carer when feeding • Becomes excited and reacts to familiar sounds; enjoys routine bathing and cares • Becomes excited with play, e.g. tickling and being babble-talked at • By 6 months everything goes into the mouth • At 6 months uses two hands to try to grasp small objects; will pass them from hand to hand and gaze at them • May be starting to show some anxiety with strangers by 6 months

Table 6.3 Normal growth and development of the infant at 9–12 months.

Posture and gross motor movements	Vision and fine motor movements
• Can sit without support and reach for objects and by 12 months can sit up from a lying down position • Can roll over on the floor, then crawl on knees and then on feet by 12 months • Can pull himself/herself up but falls down again, progressing to walking around pieces of furniture to walking aided or unaided by 12 months	• Takes more interest in objects with careful regard and moves object from hand to hand as well as turning it over • Will look at an object before attempting to grasp it, using one hand to grasp • Points and pokes at objects with index finger • Picks up small objects between thumb and index finger (pincer grasp); by 12 months uses tip of finger in neater technique • Drops objects but does not place them down; by 12 months throws toys • Can look in the right place when objects are dropped; by 12 months knows where to look if out of sight • Will carefully watch activities a few metres away for a few minutes and by 12 months further away • By 12 months may use one hand in preference to the other • May start holding and banging objects together by 12 months • At 12 months starting to look at pictures

Hearing and speech	Social behaviour and play
• Uses voice for communication shouts to call attention and listens for response before shouting again • Babbles (using repetitive sounds) at length, e.g. 'dada' to amuse self and to communicate pleasure • Understands the meaning of some words, e.g. 'goodbye' ('bobeye') and 'no' • Starting to imitate sounds, e.g. cough • Starting to localise more faint sounds • By 12 months will respond to own name • Starting to understand the meaning of more words, e.g. 'car', and commands, e.g. 'Give that to dad', at 12 months • May demonstrate understanding by imitating, e.g. brushing hair	• When feeding may hold bottle or breast • Will take, hold, bite and chew small pieces of food and by 12 months will hold cup • By 12 months will hold spoon but will make a mess of trying to eat with it • If annoyed will vocalise angrily and throw body backwards and stiffen up • Knows strangers and may cling to familiar carers, hiding face; by 12 months does not like having familiar people out of sight • Plays 'peekaboo' and will try to clap hands; by 12 months waves goodbye • Shakes noisy toys and explores them • Offers objects but unable to hand them over • Looks for an object that he/she has seen being partially or wholly hidden • By 12 months will help with dressing by holding out foot for sock • By 12 months will put objects into a box and take them out again • Easily finds toy out of view at 12 months; will give them to adults • Finds making noise with toys pleasurable and will seek to repeat the sound by 12 months

Table 6.4 Normal growth and development of the child at 15–18 months.

Posture and gross motor movements	Vision and fine motor movements
• Walking with balancing measures (legs apart, hands out) to starting to run with better balance by 18 months; may have problems negotiating any objects in the way • Can get up the stairs, progressing to getting up and down stairs by 18 months • Kneels and then squats to pick up objects by 18 months • At 18 months climbs onto things, e.g. low chairs, can sit himself/herself down on small seats and carries objects whilst walking	• Can use both hands to grasp objects with a precise pincer movement, becoming more precise with smaller objects at 18 months • Starts to build blocks; two then three high at 18 months • Uses palmar grasp to hold pencils and scribble, may start to place crudely between finger and thumb at 18 months • More interested in looking at and touching coloured pictures; starting to turn pages at 18 months • Points at objects, demanding them • May point at interesting objects outside

Hearing and speech	Social behaviour and play
• Says between two and six recognisable words with understanding, rising to 20 by 18 months • May imitate words from sentences directed at him/her at 18 months • Can point to objects when asked to, e.g. 'Point to the cow' • Will understand some simple instructions, e.g. 'Time for tea', and will carry out simple commands by 18 months, e.g. 'Get your hat' • Speech is continual and reflects mood • Taking interest in nursery rhymes and may try joining in by 18 months	• Holds spoon and takes it to mouth but turns it over until about 18 months; drinks from a cup well but may need some assistance • Helps more with dressing; starting to remove and put on some clothes by 18 months • Explores more objects and rooms; very curious – will push buttons on TV, etc. by 18 months • Carries objects by any means, e.g. doll's hair • Needs reassurance from carer as can be emotionally labile; even by 18 months likes to be alone yet needs to be able to see carer • By 18 months may start to be aware of toilet needs; may point to soiled nappies • No sense of danger and no longer puts everything into mouth by 18 months • May start to imitate household chores by about 18 months, e.g. sweeping the floor

Table 6.5 Normal growth and development of the child at 2–2¹/₂ years.

Posture and gross motor movements	Vision and fine motor movements
• Runs, avoids objects in the way and can stop easily • Can get up from squatting without using hands • Pushes and pulls things around easily • Walks up and down stairs • Can throw a ball without falling over; by 2¹/₂ can kick a ball albeit ineffectively • Pushes self along with feet when sitting on bike • By 2¹/₂ can jump down from small step with two feet together and can stand or tiptoes	• Picks up objects easily and can place them down again • Building blocks may be up to seven high • Holds pencil more correctly and may draw in a circular fashion as well as just to and fro; will try to imitate other shapes, developing to horizontal lines and some letters, e.g. t and v by 2¹/₂, often by copying • Can turn the pages one at a time in a book and increasingly recognising details in the pictures • Does not yet recognise self in photos, but by 2¹/₂, if shown, will know self in photo

Hearing and speech	Social behaviour and play
• Uses up to 50 words now and up to 200 by 2¹/₂; simple sentences with two words or more are vocalised • Talks to self more and calls self by name; may have long incomprehensible conversations with self developing into more comprehensible conversations by 2¹/₂ • Will ask names of objects and people on a constant basis; joins in singing • Can name familiar objects and hand familiar objects to carer • Likes having stories read to them by 2¹/₂	• Will ask for a drink or food; can feed self but becomes easily distracted • By 2¹/₂ may be using a fork • Starting to verbalise the need to go to the toilet but not always on time; by 2¹/₂ may be pulling down own pants (but not up again) • Becoming even more curious about environment and will run around in it; may follow carer around the house and garden • Demanding attention, having tantrums and clinging alternately; can be easily distracted, but this becomes less easy by 2¹/₂ • Knows own possessions and will defend these • Will play in presence of other children but not with them (parallel play) or share toys • If other children receive attention, may be resentful • Will start to act out roles at 2, developing these further by 2¹/₂, e.g. putting dolls in prams, mowing the lawn

Table 6.6 Normal growth and development of the 3-year-old child.

Posture and gross motor movements	Vision and fine motor movements
• Climbs more easily • Can easily avoid objects when running, pushing and pulling objects • Uses the pedals when sitting on a bike • Can stand and walk on tiptoe as well as stand on one foot • Throws a ball overhand and is starting to be able to catch a ball with arms outstretched • Can kick a ball with greater force	• Builds blocks to 10 high and maybe some bridges by $3\frac{1}{2}$ • Uses pencil with good control; copies letters and numbers; draws person with head and maybe one or two other features • May know colours • May enjoy painting pictures • Can cut paper with scissors

Hearing and speech	Social behaviour and play
• Speech has a range of loudness and tone and can communicate with strangers • Can state name and possibly age • Can explain some past experiences but mostly converses about the present • Still asking lots of questions, e.g. who, what, why • Has favourite stories and requests them over again; knows nursery rhymes and may sing them for you • May count up to ten but understands numbers up to two or three	• Eats with fork and spoon • Can pull pants up as well now • Needs help with buttons • May be dry through the night • Can wash hands but not dry them • Starts to be more affectionate and may confide in carer • Likes to help with household chores • Make-believe play can be vivid • Starting to share and play with other children • Starting to understand past, present and future

professionals must be referred for appropriate assessment and management as early as possible (Illingworth 1992). Children are a vulnerable group in society (UNICEF 1989) and together with their family have the right for the highest standard of care.

Some children miss out stages of development, e.g. go from sitting to standing without crawling, whilst others develop differently according to physical and emotional health states. A prematurely born baby may sit supported early but delay in

Table 6.7 Normal growth and development of the 4-year-old child.

Posture and gross motor movements	Vision and fine motor movements
• Can run up and down stairs • Climbs higher objects, e.g. ladders • Rides a bike (three-wheeler) easily • Can hop on one foot and stand longer on one foot • Can bend at the waist to pick up objects from the floor • Throwing, catching and kicking a ball is more effective; can use a bat	• Can build towers of up to ten blocks and several bridges; can imitate block-steps • Can spread fingers and bring thumb to each finger bilaterally when shown • Holds and uses a pencil more like an adult and can copy more symbols, e.g. v, h, t, o • Draws a person with more body parts including limbs and a trunk • House drawing is recognisable and can name objects before drawing • Can name four primary colours

Hearing and speech	Social behaviour and play
• Speech is more grammatically correct • Can talk about any recent events • Will be able to give full name, address and age • Continues to ask who, what, why and meanings of words • Maintains interest in long stories; can tell long stories but will mix up truth and fiction • Counts up to 20 and allocates numbers to objects as touching them up to five • Likes jokes • Knows and can sing several nursery rhymes	• Can wash and dry hands and brush teeth • Dresses and undresses except still has difficulty with laces and back buttons • A little more independent from carer • Will be impudent to carers and squabble with other children if does not get own way • Looks for other children to play with and will demonstrate alternating co-operation and antagonism; however, understands that arguments should be with words not violence • Understands sharing and taking turns • Will look after younger siblings and will get upset if other children are distressed • Developing sense of humour • More sophisticated make-believe and dress-up play • Creative with outside activities with any materials around • Appreciates past, present and future

Table 6.8 Normal growth and development of the 5-year-old child.

Posture and gross motor movements	Vision and fine motor movements
• Walks along a line • Skips on alternate feet • Can hop a few steps forward • Plays ball games skilfully	• Easily picks up and puts down small objects • Uses building blocks more complexly • Can write and copy more letters and symbols, e.g. X, L, A, C, U and a triangle • Draws a human and house with more details, including fingers and doors and windows • Spontaneously draws other pictures • Will colour-in pictures quite neatly, staying within the lines • Will count the fingers of one hand using the index finger of the other • Can match more colours

Hearing and speech	Social behaviour and play
• Good speech and likes reciting or singing songs • May act out stories that have been read to him/her, either alone or with other children • Can give more information about self, e.g. birth date • Likes puzzles and jokes	• Uses knife and fork well • Dresses and undresses • Can wash and dry hands and face but still requires help with rest of hygiene • More independent and reasoned behaviour • Needs to be reminded about tidiness but understands it • Complex and creative play including props • Has special friends and is more co-operative with other children; knows about being fair and having rules • Individual sense of humour • Starting to appreciate time in relation to daily activities • Goes to the aid of and protects siblings, pets and younger children • Will actively try to comfort other children in distress

sitting unsupported (Sheridan 1997). Development occurs when the child is interested, motivated and has playful interaction with carers.

Ask the parents/carers if there are any concerns; they are often the first to raise a concern. Then ask them about the activities outlined below. If unsure, you can ask the child or child and carer to engage in the activities or undertake activities with the neonate and infant. You will need an appropriate environment and props to observe the child in order to gain accurate information.

Tables 6.1–6.8 use the work of Mary Sheridan (1997) and are only *guidelines* on:

- posture and gross motor movements
- vision and fine motor movements
- hearing and speech
- social behaviour/play

Primitive reflexes
(Advanced skill)
Primitive reflexes:

- should be present at the appropriate age;
- should not be present longer than normal as persistence suggests poor cerebral cortical development where myelination of nerve sheaths is slow (Hockenbury 2003);
- should be symmetric;
- should not be associated with posturing or twitching.

Table 6.9 outlines the key primitive reflexes (Bukatko & Daehler 1998; Szilagyi 2003).

HISTORY
A comprehensive history provides a great deal of the information needed to develop a diagnosis. Children should also have the opportunity to express their perspective. This can be gained by spending time with the child and taking an interest in them, asking them unrelated questions and working towards asking them about why they think they are here or what they find difficult. When taking a history:

- do check that you understand what is being said as concepts can have different meanings, e.g. does blurring vision really mean double vision and does dizzy mean vertigo or light-headedness (Fuller 2000)?

Table 6.9 Primitive reflexes.

Name	Procedure	Result	Normal	Abnormal
Palmar (hand) grasp	Put your finger in hand	The hand should grasp the finger	From birth until 4 months	Absence may indicate neurological defect
Plantar (foot) grasp	Place finger on ball of foot	The toes should curl as if trying to grasp finger	From birth until 9 months	Absence may indicate spinal cord defect
Moro (startle)	Sit infant up allowing head to drop back a few degrees Or make a loud noise Or lower infant rapidly	The infant will move arms away from the body and extend them with hands open	From birth until 6 months	Absence or persistence beyond 6 months may indicate neurological disease
Asymmetric tonic neck	Place the infant supine and turn head to one side so that the jaw is over the shoulder	The infant's arm on the side of the face extends whilst the other flexes	From birth until 3 months	Absence or persistence beyond 3 months may indicate neurological disease
Positive support	Hold the infant around the chest, supporting the head. Lower down until the feet touch the surface	The infant's hips and knees extend and appear to be partial weight-bearing for a few seconds	From birth to 6 months	Absence may indicate hypotonia or flaccidity Prolonged time in extension may indicate a spasticity
Rooting	Gently stroke the corner of the mouth	The infant's mouth will open and turn towards the stimulus to suck	From birth to 4 months	Absence may indicate central nervous system disease
Sucking	Gently put finger on lips or in mouth	The infant will start to suck	From birth to 6 months	Absence may indicate neurological deficit
Babinski	Stroke the sole of the infant's foot	The infant's toes will fan out and curl	From birth up to 2 years	Absence may indicate neurological defects
Labyrinthine	Place the infant on his/her back Then place infant on stomach	The infant will extend arms and legs Then flex arms and legs	From birth until 4 months	Absence may indicate neurological disorder

Trunk incurvation (Galant)	With one hand, support the infant prone. With the other hand stroke the infant's back 1 cm from the vertebral column from shoulder to buttock	The infant will curve the spine toward the stimulus	From birth to 2 months	Absence may indicate a spinal cord lesion. Persistence after 2 months may indicate developmental delay
Placing and stepping	Hold the infant around the chest, supporting the head. Lower down so that one foot touches the surface	The infant will flex the foot and hip of that leg and step with the other. The infant will step alternately	From birth to 3 months for stepping and 9 months for placing	Absence of placing may indicate paralysis or birth by caesarian section. Absence of stepping may indicate neurological dysfunction
Landau	Hold the infant prone with one hand	The infant will lift the head and straighten the spine	From birth to 6 months	Absence may indicate inadequate muscle tone. Persistence beyond 6 months may indicate developmental delay
Parachute	Hold the infant prone and lower towards a surface	The infant will extend arms and legs	From 4 to 6 months and does not disappear	Delay may be indicative of future voluntary motor development delay
Swimming	Place the infant in water	The infant will hold breath, and arms and legs will move as if trying to swim	From birth until 5 months	Absence may indicate neurological dysfunction
Body righting	Rotate the infant's hips or shoulders	The infant will rotate the rest of the body	From 4 months to more than 12 months	Absence may indicate neurological defects and herald difficulty in posture and walking

- consider the time course: all signs expressed by the child or carer need to be determined whether or not there has been any progression of these or if the signs are intermittent or continuous; also note the details of any individual events.

Specific details of the history may include asking about details of any neurological event:

- headaches
- dizziness
- irritability or hyperactivity (Engel 1997)
- loss of consciousness
- nausea or vomiting
- seizures
- numbness or tingling
- sphincter disturbance
- sense loss

PHYSICAL ASSESSMENT

The neurological examination consists of examining the motor system, co-ordination, sensory system and the cranial nerves. Much of the examination can take place alongside the musculo-skeletal assessment (Engel 1997). The cranial nerves are discussed in Chapter 11. The following text outlines techniques available for use to assess the neurological system, followed by a section on their application to different age groups.

MOTOR SYSTEM

Upper motor neurones (UMN) (direct pathways also known as pyramidal tracts; and indirect pathways also known as extrapyramidal tracts) extend from the brain (cortex or brainstem) to the lower motor neurones (Tortora & Grabowski 2003). Muscle weakness from UMN defects are demonstrated with:

- increased tone
- increased reflexes
- weak extension in the arms
- weak flexion in the legs (Fuller 2000).

The basal ganglia and cerebellum influence the upper motor neurones by receiving sensory, associative and motor information from the cortex and then sending feedback to the motor cortex via the thalamus. This works by initiating and terminating movements (Tortora & Grabowski 2003), e.g. starting and stopping walking.

Lower motor neurones (LMN) extend out of the brainstem and spinal cord to innervate skeletal muscles in the head and body. Muscle weakness from LMN defects are demonstrated with:

- wasting
- fasciculation
- decreased tone
- absent reflexes (Fuller 2000).

However, neuromuscular junction weakness is demonstrated with:

- a tiring weakness
- normal or decreased tone
- normal reflexes (Fuller 2000).

Physical examination includes the following (note: asterisks indicate those examinations used in neurological screening for young people – see below, 'The Young Person').

Inspection*
(Basic skill)
Observe the body position at rest and on movement. Note any:

- asymmetries;
- tripping, clumsiness (cerebellum regulates posture and balance);
- involuntary movements (basal ganglia and cerebellum responsible for subconscious skeletal muscle movements), e.g. tremors, tics, fasciculation.

Bulk*
(Basic skill)
Observe and palpate all major muscles to determine appropriate size of muscles (muscle wastage may indicate damage to neurological pathways):

- hands, shoulders, thighs, calves
- symmetry muscle bulk – check for symmetrical as well as proximal/distal appropriateness.

Tone*
(Advanced skill)
Normally there is slight tension of muscles even when they are relaxed (basal ganglia and brainstem are responsible for tone). Try to get the child to be as relaxed as possible and put all limbs through a range of movements, all the while feeling for the normal tone. Hold the hand or foot with one hand and the knee or elbow with the other, flex and extend the arm/leg and rotate gently at the shoulder/hip. Note any:

- decreased resistance or floppiness, which may indicate
  - abnormalities of the peripheral nervous system (lower motor neurones) or cerebellum
  - acute spinal cord injury
- increased resistance, jerkiness or spasticity, which may indicate an upper motor neurone abnormality.

Strength
(Advanced skill)
Strength involves testing power.

- Ask the child to move against your resistance or resist your movement, push against or pull a toy.
- Generalised weakness could be due to nerve, muscular or neuromuscular damage.
- Symmetrical proximal muscle weakness may suggest a myopathy.
- Symmetrical weakness of distal muscles may suggest a peripheral nerve abnormality (Dooley 1997).
- Upper motor neurone (pyramidal) weakness usually affects finger extension, elbow extension and shoulder abduction, hip flexion, knee flexion and foot dorsiflexion.
- Lower motor neurone weakness usually presents as a generalised weakness (Fuller 2000).

The following tests show the associated muscle, nerve and root (in parentheses) (Fuller 2000; Bickley 2003):

- *arm flexion (biceps – musculocutaneous nerve – C5/C6) and extension (triceps – radial nerve – C6/C7/C8)
  - Ask the child to bend arms in front of him/her.
  - Have the child pull and push against your hand (Engel 1997).
- wrist extension (radial nerve – C6/C7/C8)
  - Ask the child to make a fist and resist you pushing it downwards.
  - Weakness may indicate peripheral nerve damage or central nervous system hemiplegia.
- hand grip (C7/C8/T1)
  - Ask the child to grip and squeeze two of your fingers and not let go (Engel 1997).
  - Cross your fingers so it does not hurt so much.
  - Do both hands together.
  - Try to remove your fingers.
  - A weak grip may indicate either a peripheral or central nervous abnormality.
- *finger abduction (first dorsal interosseous – ulnar nerve – C8/T1)
  - Ask the child to spread fingers with palms facing down.
  - Ask the child not to let you push the fingers together.
  - Try to push fingers together by pushing index and little finger towards each other.
  - A weakness suggests ulnar nerve disorder.
- *thumb opposition (abductor pollicis brevis – median nerve – C8/T1)
  - Ask the child to try to touch his or her little finger with the thumb.
  - The examiner tries to prevent this using his/her index finger pulling against the thumb.
  - A weakness suggests median nerve disorder, e.g. carpal tunnel syndrome.
- flexion, extension and lateral bending of the spine
  - Ask the child to bend forward and backwards.
  - Ask the child to bend laterally, trying to touch the knee with the hand.

- chest expansion in respiration (see Chapter 2)
- hip – the child can sit on the edge of the bed for this
  - *flexion (iliopsoas – lumbar sacral plexus – L2/L3/L4): ask the child to push his/her thighs up against your hand as you push down on the thigh;
  - extension (gluteus maximus – inferior gluteal nerve – S1): ask the child to push his/her thighs down on your hand as you push upwards on the posterior thigh;
  - adduction (adductors – obdurator nerve – L2/L3/L4): ask the child to try to close his/her legs together and push against your hands which are placed between the child's thighs.
  - abduction (gluteus medius and mimimus – superior gluteal nerve – L4/L5/S1): ask the child to try to spread his/her legs and push against your hands as you place them outside the child's knees.
- knee
  - *flexion (hamstrings – sciatic nerve – L4/L5/S1/S2): ask the child to sit on the edge of a bed and to push against your hands as you push against the shinbones;
  - *extension (quadriceps – femoral nerve – L2/L3/L4): ask the child to sit on the edge of the bed and to push against your hands as you pull the calves forward.
- ankle
  - *dorsiflexion (tibialis anterior – deep peroneal nerve – L4/L5): ask the child to pull against your hand as you try to push the foot downwards;
  - *extension – plantar flexion (gastrocnemius – posterior tibial nerve – S1): ask the child to push against your hand as you try to push the ball of the foot upwards.

CO-ORDINATION

Co-ordination requires integration of the:

- motor system (including basal ganglia);
- cerebellar system for rhythmic/fine movement and posture;
- vestibular system for balance and eye/head/body co-ordination;

- sensory system for position sense (part of proprioception – knowing where our limbs are and their movement even if we are not looking at them).

Co-ordination can be tested by the following methods.

Rapid alternating movements
(Advanced skill)

These may be impaired by cerebellar disease, upper motor neurone weakness or basal ganglia disease:

- Hand slaps: show the child how to slap the thigh with the hand, lift up the hand and turn it over and slap the thigh again with the back of the hand; ask them to repeat this as fast as possible.
- Index finger to thumb distal interphalangeal (DIP) joint: show the child how to tap the DIP joint with the tip of the index finger; repeat as rapidly as possible: the dominant side will normally do better.
- Ball of foot slaps: ask the child to tap your hand with the ball of the child's feet (one at a time) as fast as the child can; usually not done as well as hands (Bickley 2003).

Point-to-point testing
(Advanced skill)

These exercises may be impaired by cerebellar disease:

- Arms
    - *Nose to finger: ask the child to use his/her index finger to touch the nose and then your finger several times; move your finger about a little so that direction is changed and occasional extension is required by the child; note any tremors.
    - Hold your finger so that the child can touch it with his/her index finger with arm outstretched; ask the child to lift his/her hand above his/her head and then bring it down to touch your finger again; do this several times with eyes open and then with eyes closed (loss of position sense is suggested if there is inaccuracy with eyes closed).

- Legs
  - *Heel slide: ask the child to put the heel of one foot on the knee of the other leg and then slide it down the leg to the toes with eyes open (to test cerebellar function) and then with eyes closed (to test position sense) (Bickley 2003).

Gait*
(Normal gait observation is a basic skill; the rest of the gait techniques are advanced skills)

- Observe normal gait as the child enters the room – check symmetry, arm swing, size of paces.
- Heel/toe (tandem walking): ask the child to walk in a straight line putting one foot immediately in front of the other in a heel-to-toe fashion (may reveal ataxia).
- Heels: ask the child to walk on the heels:
  - inability to heel walk is a sensitive test for corticospinal tract weakness; there may be a muscular weakness in toes or heels
- Tiptoes: ask the child to walk on the toes.
- Hop: in place one foot at a time:
  - inability may indicate weakness, loss of position sense or cerebellar defect.
- Knee bends: one side then the other:
  - inability suggests weakness of muscles.
- Stance: always stand close to the child in case the child looks like he/she will fall:
  - *Romberg*: the child stands with feet together and then closes eyes for 20–30 seconds. Inability to maintain position suggests loss of position sense (part of proprioception).
  - **Pronator drift*: the child stands with legs together (or sits) and holds arms stretched out horizontally palm up and eyes closed for 20–30 seconds. If pronation occurs (hand turns over), it suggests a contralateral lesion in the corticospinal tract.

Then tap the arms so that they bounce downward; watch for them to bounce back to original position:
- a weak arm will stay pushed down;
- with loss of position sense, the child may not know the arm is out of line;
- with cerebellar problems, the arm will bounce back but will overshoot (Bickley 2003).

Reflexes*
(Advanced skill)
(1) Primitive: (see above 'Normal growth and development').
(2) Deep tendon – stretch reflexes cause contraction of skeletal muscles in response to stretching of the tendon; must have intact sensory and motor neuron pathways as well as intact neuromuscular junction. Table 6.10 shows the reflexes to be tested.
- Use different strategies to get the child as relaxed as possible:
  - ask child to close eyes;
  - distract with a toy or game;
  - tell a story or get the child to tell you a story.
- Position the limbs as accurately as possible.
- When striking the tendon, do it as briskly, quickly and directly as possible.
- Compare sides.
- Note the response:

$$2+ = \text{brisk (normal)}$$
$$1+ = \text{diminished}$$
$$0 = \text{no response}$$

A hyperactive response suggests a central nervous system problem (upper motor neurone) and if there is a sustained clonus (rhythmic movements) and positive Babinski, this will confirm it. A decreased response may be due to:
- lost sensation
- correlating spinal segments damaged
- peripheral nerve damage
- diseases of the muscles or deficits in the neuromuscular junction (e.g. paralysing agents).

Table 6.10 Reflex testing (Engel 1997; Bickley 2003).

Reflexes	Examination techniques
Biceps Look for flexion of the arm and feel for muscle contraction	Slightly bend the arm and place the palm downwards and resting on the child's lap (or abdomen if lying down) Lay your finger or thumb across the cubital fossa and with the pointed aspect of the hammer strike the examiner's finger
Triceps Look for slight extension of the arm	Flex the arm at the elbow and hold the arm in this position with the child's hand prone on his/her lap (or across the chest if lying down), or hold the arm laterally in the air at 90°, supporting the arm at the cubital fossa Strike the tendon with the pointed aspect of the hammer just above the elbow
Brachioradialis Look for flexion and palm turning upward	Lay the child's hand, ulnar surface resting on his/her lap (or abdomen if lying down) and lightly hold the wrist Strike the tendon with the blunt aspect of the hammer about 1–2 inches above the wrist
Abdominal Look for contraction of the abdominal muscles and the umbilicus deviating toward the stimulus	Expose the child's abdomen Stroke the abdomen from the distal quadrants, one at a time, towards the umbilicus with a cotton-tip
Knees Look for lower leg extension and feel for muscle contraction	Flex the knee by asking the child to sit on the edge of a chair with legs dangling (or bending the leg and supporting the knee if the child is lying supine) Gently hold the quadriceps muscles and tap the patellar tendon just below the patella with the sharp aspect of the hammer
Achilles' Look for and feel plantar flexion at the ankle	With the child sitting (if the child is lying down, place the ankle to be examined on the shin of the other leg), pull the toes upward, thereby dorsiflexing the foot at the ankle Strike the Achilles' tendon just above the heel with the blunt aspect of the hammer

Table 6.10 *Continued.*

Reflexes	Examination techniques
Plantar Look for the toes flexing	With the child sitting or lying down (supine), stroke (as lightly as will stimulate a response) the lateral aspect of the sole of the foot from the heel to the little toe and then across the ball of the foot with the wooden end of a cotton-tip or thumbnail Babinski response is normal in children less than 2 years but may suggest a central nervous system lesion in the corticospinal tract (upper motor neurone lesion) or in the post-ictal period after a seizure in older children
Cremasteric Testes retract into inguinal canal	Stroke upper inner thigh
Clonus Look and feel for rhythmic movements	Partly flex the knee and support it with one hand, while with the other, dorsiflex then plantar flex the foot a few times, finishing with a sharp dorsiflex and holding it there Sustained clonus (foot dorsiflexes and plantar flexes repeatedly and rhythmically) indicates upper motor neurone disease (more than four flex/dorsiflex movements)

SENSORY SYSTEM
(Advanced skills)
Sensory impulses travel via the:

- spinal nerves and their branches, spinal cord, then to brainstem
  - via the spinothalamic tract or posterior column, and then to the primary somatosensory area in the cerebral cortex
  - via the spinocerebellar tract and then to the cerebellum
- cranial nerves (Tortora & Grabowski 2003).

The following tests establish normal transmission of sensation; any anomalies could be due to damage to any part of the pathway. Test where there is history of numbness, motor or reflex abnormalities. Sensory mapping will help to establish the level of block in a spinal injury or if epidural blocks are being used for pain management. A knowledge of dermatones and peripheral nerve paths is essential. Always compare symmetry:

- loss of sensation on one side is due to a spinal cord or higher pathway lesion;
- bilateral distal sensory loss indicates a polyneuropathy (affecting several nerves).

Do your best not to use a set pattern or pace for testing as the patient may pick this up. With pain, temperature and touch, compare proximal and distal sensations.

Sample different dermatones and include:

- shoulders (C4)
- outer and inner forearms (C6/T1)
- thumbs and little fingers (C6/C8)
- anterior thighs (L2)
- calves: medial and lateral (L4/L5)
- little toe (S1)

With each of these tests, *always* show the child what you will do before doing it and check that the child understands what he/she has to do (Bickley 2003).

Pain and temperature*

These exercises test the spinothalamic tracts.

- Use a sharp but safe tool such as a 'neurological pin'; one end should be blunt and the other sharp; apply the tool to the child, alternating (on an irregular basis) sharp and dull.
- Ask the child to close eyes and respond to touch by stating whether the stimulus is sharp or dull.
- If there is any doubt over the response, it may be useful to use a hot and cold response; two test-tubes – one filled with hot water and the other cold – can be applied, asking the child to identify either hot or cold (Bickley 2003).

Light touch*

These exercises test the spinothalamic tracts and posterior column pathway.

- Using a little cotton wool, ask the child to close eyes and respond when he/she can feel the cotton wool; make sure you only 'dab' the cotton wool on the skin.
- Use cotton wool to make symmetrical and proximal/distal comparisons; ask the child, 'Does this (dab) feel like this (dab in another area to compare symmetry or proximal/distal)?'.

Vibration*

These exercises test the posterior column pathway. Test fingers and toes and if these are normal, assume that any proximal measures will be normal; if abnormal responses are found, move proximally up to the next bony prominence, e.g. wrist or malleolus.

- Set a tuning fork in motion, ask the child to close eyes and place it over the distal interphalangeal (DIP) joint of the finger and big toe.
- Take care to hold the tuning fork in the correct position; if you hold it too high, the vibration will be interfered with.
- Ask the child what he/she feels; if the child is not sure, then ask him/her to tell you when 'it' stops; reach up and stop the vibration by squeezing with thumb and finger without any movement of the tuning fork; you may need to hold the tuning fork and DIP with one hand, leaving the free hand to stop the vibration. Often vibration is the first sensation lost in peripheral neuropathy (Bickley 2003).

Position* (proprioception)

These exercises test the posterior column pathway. Test fingers and toes and if these are normal, assume that any proximal measures will be normal; if abnormal responses are found, move proximally to the wrist or ankle.

- Ask the child to either sit or lie down and to close eyes.
- Hold the big toe at the sides of the toe with your thumb and index finger; manoeuvre it away from the other toes.
- Move the toe joint up and down several times one side then the other, taking care not to have a set pattern.
- Ask the child to say whether the movement is 'up' or 'down' (Bickley 2003).

Discrimination

These exercises test the posterior column pathways. Ask the child to close his/her eyes before each test.

- *Stereognosis*
  - o Place a familiar object in the child's hand; ask the child to identify the object.
- *Two-point discrimination*
  - o Using a paperclip (which has been unfolded and bent so that two prongs are able to be pressed to the skin simultaneously) with the two points 10 mm apart, press both prongs into the side of the child's index finger and ask the child whether he/she can feel one or two pricks.
  - o Then prod the skin with a single prong; ask the child if he/she can feel one or two pricks.
  - o Continue the exercise, each time narrowing the width between the double prong and alternating with a single prong; ask the child to tell you if he/she can feel one prick or two; when the double prong becomes less than 5 mm apart, it will feel like one prick.
- *Point localisation*
  - o Briefly touch the child on the trunk and legs, one random place at a time, and ask the child each time to open eyes and point to where you touched.
- *Extinction*
  - o Simultaneously touch the child on two symmetrical parts of the trunk and legs, randomly; ask the child to point to where you touched (Fuller 2000).

ASSESSING THE INFANT

Neurological disease is suspected if any of the following is found:

- unusual irritability
- posture asymmetrical
- extension of head, neck and extremities
- floppiness
- decreased response to pain

Dysmorphic features may suggest a syndrome (Dooley 1997).

Inspect and assess
(Basic skill)
- head circumference
- presence of cranial bruit (see Chapter 11)
- fontanelles (see Chapter 11)

Motor tone and strength
(Observation is a basic skill; the rest are advanced skills)
- Observe position at rest: (normally flexed)
  - there may be a normal slight tremor in the newborn
  - neck extension may occur with cerebral irritation (Gill & O'Brien 2002).
- Test resistance to passive movement.
- Manipulate each major joint through its full range of movement and note any spasticity or flaccidity.
- Grasp the infant's hands and pull gently forward to a sitting position; the head flexes and should hold momentarily when upright (Gill & O'Brien 2002); repeat in 24 hours if there is a head lag (indicates hypotonia).
- Hold the infant under the arms and hold in a vertical position; the infant should support self but if he/she slips through grip, hypotonia is evident (Gill & O'Brien 2002).
- Place the infant face down on the palm of your hand and note the back extending, arms and legs flexing, hips extending with the head lifting and rotating; a 'rag doll' stance implies a hypotonia (Gill & O'Brien 2002).
- Hypotonia may be caused by a muscle weakness (lower motor neurone disease) or cerebellar lesions, neuropathies or malnutrition.
- See normal growth and development of the posture/gross and fine motor (above).

Co-ordination
See normal growth and development fine motor activities (above).

Reflexes
(1) Primitive reflexes *(advanced skill)*: see above in normal growth and development.

(2) Deep tendon reflexes (*advanced skill*):
- The examiner may substitute an index or middle finger for the hammer (Gill & O'Brien 2002).
- The response can be indeterminate and variable as corticospinal pathways are not fully developed.
- Before the age of 6 months the triceps, brachioradialis and abdominal reflexes are difficult to get a response from (Szilagyi 2003).
- The anal reflex is present at birth and should be tested by a health care practitioner (check to see who is the most appropriate person to do this in your practice, e.g. medical staff or nurse practitioner). This checks for spinal cord lesion, e.g. spina bifida.
  - Lie the baby prone or lateral and part the buttocks gently.
  - Stroke the anal margin/perianal area lightly with a cotton tip.
  - The external anal sphincter should briskly contract (Engel 1997).
- When testing the plantar reflex, note that a positive Babinski sign is normal in the child up to 2 years of age.
- There may not be a response to Achilles' tendon tapping for the ankle response but if it is important to assess, then grasping the infant's malleolus with one hand and abruptly dorsiflexing the ankle may produce a response. A further response may include up to ten normal clonus beats (Szilagyi 2003).

Sensory
(Advanced skill)
This is limited; you can check for pain sensation by flicking the sole or hand and note withdrawal, arousal and change in facial expression, but you should only do this if you have concerns. Absence of sensation may be noted through flaccidity, e.g. a myelomeningocoele or Guillain-Barré syndrome (Gill & O'Brien 2002).

THE PRE-SCHOOL CHILD
It is important to try to distinguish between a developmental delay and a neurological problem. Try to have fun with the child

to enhance co-operation. At this age, children are probably wanting to show you what they can do.

Inspect and assess
Motor tone and strength
(Observation is a basic skill; the rest are advanced skills)
- Observe the child when entering the room and during consultation.
- Note asymmetries, weakness, tripping or clumsiness.
  - Remember that normal gait is usually a little clumsy when first starting to walk.
  - A child with a hemiplegia may not want to use the affected limb at all.
- Gower's sign may be seen in muscular dystrophy, where the child stands by rolling to prone position and pushing self up off the floor with arms and extended legs.
- Test upper arm strength by holding the child's legs while he/she puts arms extended to the ground and pretends to do a 'wheelbarrow' race (Dooley 1997).
- See normal growth and development of the posture/gross and fine motor activities (above).

Co-ordination
(Advanced skills except normal growth and development)
- Hand preference is not obvious before 18 months.
- You can do some rapid alternating movements, including finger–nose exercise.
- Carry out heel–toe walking and hopping.
- If the child is constantly unsteady with frequent falling and dropping objects, ataxia is indicated.
- The 'waddling' child with a proximal weakness may have muscular dystrophy (Dooley 1997).
- Hemiplegia will be evidenced by dragging the affected limb and not using it (Gill & O'Brien 2002).
- See normal growth and development of fine motor activities (above).
- Orthopaedic causes of poor gait need differentiating from neurological defects such as cerebral palsy, ataxia, neuromuscular or degenerative disease.

Reflexes
(Advanced skill)
- Get the child to close eyes to help relax.
- Let the child use and play with the hammer first; convince the child that it will not hurt.

Sensory
(Advanced skill)
- Use cotton wool and ask when it 'tickles', but do not use sharp tools (the child will not like it).

THE SCHOOL-AGE CHILD
Note that children will often try to please you and so they might look to give you the answers that they think you want rather than what is really happening.

Inspect and assess
Inspect and assess using many of the techniques outlined above.

Motor tone and strength
(Observation is a basic skill; the rest are advanced skills)
- Observe the child when entering the room and during consultation.
- Observe ability to write, draw, kick and catch a ball.
- Test pelvic girdle (proximal) strength by asking child to arise from supine without using arms or do deep knee bends (Dooley 1997).
- Weakness and wasting of hand muscles indicate neuropathy.
- A limb with increased tone may be held in an unusual position – look at wear pattern on shoes (Dooley 1997).

Co-ordination
(Observation is a basic skill; the rest are advanced skills)
- Gait can be assessed by observing a dance or skipping (ask the child what he/she likes doing); can the child walk a straight line heel to toe, hop, walk on tiptoes or heels, or stand on one leg?

- Heel walking will show a weakness in dorsiflexion of the foot, indicating early peripheral neuropathy (Dooley 1997).
- Romberg: the child can stand with one foot in front of the other.
- Ask the child to show you how he/she ties shoe laces or buttons a shirt.
- Ask the child to do a puzzle.
- The child can do some rapid alternating movements and point-to-point testing.
- The 'piroutte test' involves the child doing three 360° turns while walking. Alternatively ask the child to walk around a chair; a child with cerebellar disease will stumble toward the side of the lesion (Dooley 1997).

Reflexes
(Advanced skills)
- Abnormal movements may suggest cerebral palsy.
- Get the child to close eyes to help relax.
- You must let the child use and play with the hammer first; convince the child that it will not hurt.

Sensory
(Advanced skills)
- Light touch sensory tests can be used.
- Stereognosis and point localisation can be performed.
- Vibration and position sense can also be tested (Dooley 1997).

THE YOUNG PERSON
If the history suggests no neurological deficit and you can detect no speech or higher function deficit, those tests outlined above and marked with an asterisk will provide a screening neurological examination; any abnormalities detected indicate further testing (Fuller 2000).

When undertaking reflex testing, the young person can be asked to:

- clench teeth (for upper limb reflex response);
- cup fingers and lock them together in front of the body, pulling (to reinforce lower limb reflex responses).

Case Study

Mary is a 6-year-old girl who has been admitted to the children's ward with weakness in her lower limbs. She had 'flu-like' symptoms about a month ago which resolved after a week or so. She has a differential diagnosis of Guillain-Barré syndrome. Her growth and development assessment shows that she is 115 cm in height and 20 kg in weight. Her hearing, speech, vision, social behaviour and play, and fine motor movements of her upper limbs show normal patterns.

Mary's neurological examination shows:

Motor tone and strength

- Slow in walking and clumsy when trying to kick a ball but able to catch the ball.
- Muscle bulk in all four limbs appears normal.
- Decreased tone in lower limbs; normal in upper limbs.
- Normal muscle strength except reduced dorsiflexion and extension of ankle, and slight weakness in flexion and extension of the knee.

Reflexes

	Biceps	Triceps	Brachio-radialis	Patellar	Achilles'
Right	2+	2+	2+	1+	0
Left	2+	2+	2+	1+	0

Co-ordination

- Cannot heel walk, walk on tip toes, stand on one leg, skip or hop.
- It can be tested by rapid alternating movements (RAMS) in upper limbs and point-to-point intact.
- Romberg negative.

Sensory

- Light touch, vibration and position sense intact in upper limbs and lower limbs above the ankle.

- Stereognosis intact.
- Point localisation intact in upper body and lower limbs above the ankles.

Cranial nerves

- Nerves I–XII intact.

SUMMARY

Neurological assessment in the infant and child is challenging. Normal growth and development is varied in children and this can impact on the assessment. The health care practitioner needs to determine which tests are required. A screening test can be used in young people. Health care practitioners need to work closely with the parents or carers to understand and interpret findings more accurately.

REFERENCES

Bickley, L.S. (2003) *Bates Guide to Physical Examination and History Taking*, 8th edn. Lippincott, Williams and Wilkins, Philadelphia, Chapters 15, 16 and 17.

Bukatko, D. & Daehler, M.W. (1998) *Child Development: A Thematic Approach*, 3rd edn. Houghton Mifflin, Boston.

Dooley, J.M. (1997) Pediatric neurologic examination. In: Goldbloom, R.B. (ed) *Pediatric Clinical Skills*, 2nd edn. Churchill Livingston, Philadelphia, pp 259–287.

Engel, J. (1997) *Pediatric Assessment*, 3rd edn. Mosby, St. Louis.

Fuller, G. (2000) *Neurological Examination Made Easy*, 3rd edn. Churchill Livingston, Edinburgh.

Gill, D. & O'Brien, N. (2002) *Paediatric Clinical Examination Made Easy*, 4th edn. Churchill Livingston, Edinburgh.

Illingworth, R. (1992) *The Development of the Infant and Young Child*, 9th edn. Churchill Livingston, London.

Sheridan, M.D. (1997) *From Birth to Five Years: Children's Developmental Progress*. Revised and updated by Frost, M. & Sharma, A. Routledge, London.

Szilagyi, P.G. (2003) Assessing children: infancy through adolescence. In: Bickley, L.S. (2003) *Bates Guide to Physical Examination and History Taking*, 8th edn. Lippincott, Williams and Wilkins, Philadelphia, Chapter 17.

Tortora, G.J. & Grabowski, S.R. (2003) *Principles of Anatomy and Physiology*, 10th edn. John Wiley, New York.

UNICEF (1989) *Convention on the Rights of the Child*. UN, Geneva.

Acute Neurological Assessment and Monitoring

INTRODUCTION

Behavioural changes of infants and children may herald a deteriorating clinical condition. It is therefore important that all children who are sick have their behaviour observed.

When an infant or child has sustained an acute neurological injury (including head and spinal injury), neurological assessment is important to identify a baseline of brain function and monitor any changes in condition, especially when the injury causes an increase in intracranial pressure. This is usually assessed and documented through clinical examination and the use of a tool, e.g. the Glasgow Coma Scale. NICE (2003) guidelines recommend the chart shown in Fig. 7.1.

Children who have suffered an acute injury often also require ongoing monitoring. The use of technology to help monitor and manage a child with a neurological insult requires accurate and safe techniques. The overall aim of this chapter is to understand and undertake accurate assessment and monitoring.

LEARNING OBJECTIVES

By the end of this chapter the reader will be able to:

❑ Understand the rationale for the techniques used in coma scoring.
❑ Recognise and interpret signs of raised intracranial pressure.
❑ Be able to use technology accurately and safely.

BEHAVIOUR

Although there can be a psychosocial impact of hospitalisation on the child, changes of behaviour can indicate

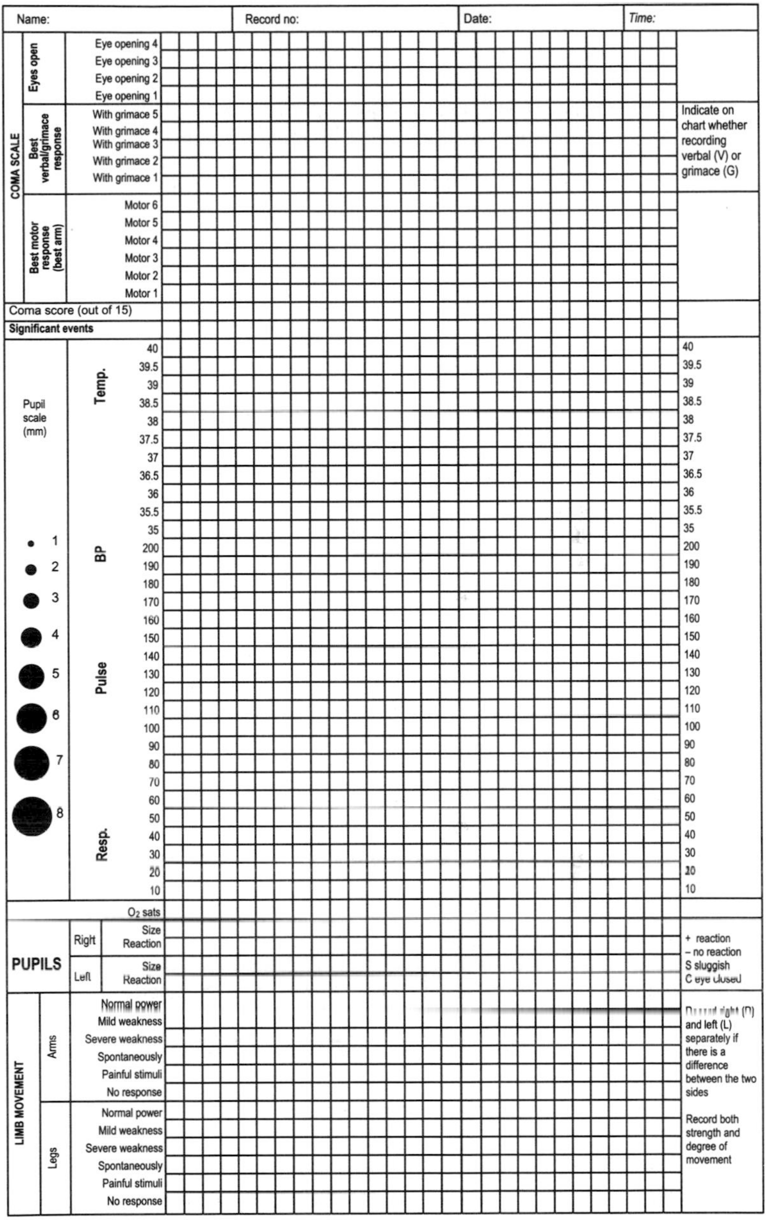

Name:	Record no:	Date:	Time:

COMA SCALE

Eyes open
- Eye opening 4
- Eye opening 3
- Eye opening 2
- Eye opening 1

Best verbal/grimace response
- With grimace 5
- With grimace 4
- With grimace 3
- With grimace 2
- With grimace 1

Indicate on chart whether recording verbal (V) or grimace (G)

Best motor response (best arm)
- Motor 6
- Motor 5
- Motor 4
- Motor 3
- Motor 2
- Motor 1

Coma score (out of 15)

Significant events

Pupil scale (mm)

Temp.
- 40
- 39.5
- 39
- 38.5
- 38
- 37.5
- 37
- 36.5
- 36
- 35.5
- 35

Pupil scale:
- 1
- 2
- 3
- 4
- 5
- 6
- 7
- 8

BP
- 200
- 190
- 180
- 170
- 160
- 150
- 140
- 130
- 120
- 110
- 100
- 90
- 80
- 70
- 60
- 50

Pulse

Resp.
- 40
- 30
- 20
- 10

O_2 sats

PUPILS

Right	Size	
	Reaction	
Left	Size	
	Reaction	

+ reaction
– no reaction
S sluggish
C eye closed

LIMB MOVEMENT

Arms
- Normal power
- Mild weakness
- Severe weakness
- Spontaneously
- Painful stimuli
- No response

Record right (R) and left (L) separately if there is a difference between the two sides

Legs
- Normal power
- Mild weakness
- Severe weakness
- Spontaneously
- Painful stimuli
- No response

Record both strength and degree of movement

Fig. 7.1 Paediatric neurological observation proforma.

cardiopulmonary and neurological compromise. Health care professionals caring for sick children must observe for the following (basic skills):

- When there is inadequate gas exchange children and infants can look tense, tired and anxious (Gill & O'Brien 2002). Tiredness can be assessed by the child's ability to speak; note how many words/sentences can be spoken and compare with normal for the child.
- Anxiety, restlessness and irritability (that cannot be attributed to tiredness, hunger, wet/dirty nappies, etc.) may indicate hypoxia.
- Drowsiness and obtundation (sleeps all the time and when stimulated responds only in a limited manner) indicate hypercapnoea.
- Lethargy is a more specific indicator of neurological compromise and can be defined as the ability to rouse to stimulation but respond in a limited way and may be disorientated (Hazinski 1992).
- The confused child is unable to think and therefore responds in an incoherent manner.
- The child whose parents/carers are concerned about 'abnormal' responses or behaviour should be assessed.

This behaviour assessment may be included as part of an early warning scoring system for sick children (Monaghan 2005).

COMA SCORING
(Basic skill)
Consciousness has two aspects that are assessed: (1) wakefulness or arousal, which is a function of the reticular activating system, and (2) cognition, a function of the cerebral hemispheres. A coma scoring system helps to identify levels of consciousness by assessing arousal (awareness of the environment) and cognition (showing that the child understands what the assessor wants through performing tasks).

This coma scoring system (based on the Glasgow Coma Score and often known as the GCS) scores from 3 to 15, with 15 being normal response. Scores below 12 require closer monitoring and below 8 indicate the need for endotracheal intubation and ventilation (NICE 2003). Abnormal GCS scores indicate that half-hourly observations should be continued (NICE 2003).

When completing your shift, undertake a set of neurological observations together with the oncoming staff to ascertain shared understanding of the documentation and promote inter-observer reliability.

Where there is developmental delay, work closely with the carers to identify normal parameters. These need detailed and careful documentation.

Begin with least noxious stimuli first and take care not to harm the child. Use dots and join these to demonstrate changes and trends in scoring (May 2001).

The three parts making up the coma scoring system are:

(1) eye opening
(2) best verbal or grimace response
(3) best motor response

Eye opening
Eye opening assesses arousal mechanisms.

- The best response is that the child opens eyes spontaneously (scores 4), but if not, determine what it takes for the eyes to open.
- First, use the patient's name to call the child in a normal voice, then repeat the call, then call in a louder voice (score 3). The child's family may help here.
- If there is no response score 2 and use painful stimuli by applying (document which one is used):
  - supra-orbital pressure with a finger (press on the groove in the bony ridge above the eye socket) except when facial trauma is present;
  - trapezius muscle pinch (pinch the muscle between the head and shoulders and twist slightly) for children over 5 years old;
  - a sternal rub (clench fist and rub centre of sternum with knuckles) except when chest trauma is present; this is not always considered best practice as localising, noted by movement of the arm up to the level of the jaw, may not be ascertained;

- o nail bed squeeze (using finger and thumb squeeze the nail bed of fingers and toes). This technique is not recommended and not best practice as it can give a spinal response rather than a central response (Hickey 2003) and cause damage to the nail bed;
- o the side of the finger can be used; place the length of a pencil against the side of the finger near the tip and exert pressure by pushing the pencil against the finger both above and below the finger tip. This technique may elicit a spinal response rather than a central response.
- • If there is no response at all, score 1.

Best verbal or grimace response
This determines cognition and awareness.

- • Verbal response of a young person/older child: ask patient his or her name, where he/she is, what school he/she goes to.
  - o The best response (score V5) is when the child can answer appropriately.
  - o If the child provides a confusing or inappropriate answer, score V4.
  - o Where there is inappropriate speech or words unrelated to conversation, score V3.
  - o Where speech is unintelligible (e.g. babbling), score V2.
  - o If there is no response, score V1.
- • Verbal response of a younger child/infant: stand close to the patient and carry out a short developmental-appropriate dialogue, e.g. babbling, simple words/sentences.
  - o The best response (score V5) is when the child appears alert, babbles, smiles or responds with simple words which are developmentally appropriate.
  - o Where there is an irritable cry or decreased normal response, score V4.
  - o If crying or screaming is exhibited that is not appropriate, score V3.
  - o Any grunting or moaning scores V2.
  - o No response scores V1.
- • Grimace: where the child is unable to verbalise (e.g. a child is intubated, an infant less than 8 months old) a verbal

response is not possible and therefore the grimace score can be used (Warren 2000). However, it must be noted that the grimace score measures different areas of cerebral function. Facial or oro-motor responses evoked by a stimulation are recorded.

- o The best response (score G5) is when a facial or mouthing activity is seen spontaneously or with developmental-appropriate voice stimulation (see above in verbal response).
- o If there is no response to verbal stimuli or response only to light touch, then score G4.
- o If there is no response, apply painful stimuli (as above) and score G3 if there is a vigorous response.
- o Score G2 if there is a mild response.
- o Score G1 if there is no response to painful stimuli.

Best motor response

This determines if the patient is aware of his or her environment, and understands and carries out tasks as instructed. According to normal and appropriate developmental ability:

- Ask the child to undertake an activity, e.g. lift up arm, push your hand, squeeze finger (and let go).
- Note normal spontaneous movements in the infant.
  - o Score 6 for normal responses.
  - o Apply painful stimuli (as above) and score 5
    - – if the child localises to the pain (localising means that the child has received the sensory stimulation and then acts to push the cause of the pain away by bringing a hand up to above chin level to push you away from undertaking supra-orbital pressure or trapezius pinch). Note that other activities may give you the information you need without continually performing these stimuli, e.g. the child pulling an oxygen mask off or pushing you away when attempting to place a naso-gastric tube (Shah 1999). Precise localisation may be less effective in the young child (May 2001).
    - – if the infant withdraws to touch.

- o If the child/infant tries to move away from the painful stimuli, or flexes arm towards the source of pain (but not acting to push away), score 4.
- o Abnormal flexion or 'decorticate movement' occurs with dysfunction of the cortex and damage to cortical-spinal nerve pathways. The child flexes arm, and rotates the wrist in a spastic posture. The legs become rigid with feet extending. Score 3 if this occurs (poor outcome).
- o Abnormal extension or 'decerebrate movement' occurs with dysfunction of the cortex and brainstem at brainstem level. The child will extend the arms and rotate them inwards and the legs become rigid and extend. Score 2 if this occurs (poor outcome).
- o Score 1 if there is no response to painful stimuli.

OTHER ASSESSMENT INFORMATION REQUIRED
Although the coma score provides an indication of the neurological status of the child further information is required to assist with decision-making.

Assessment of limb movement
There are four assessments to be made: two for arms and two for legs.

- First, all four limbs are assessed for power by the patient's ability to overcome applied resistance:
  - o Ask the patient to push or pull each arm and leg toward or away from you as you apply resistance. According to normal development the child should be able to make a good effort to do this.
  - o One (or both) side(s) may be weaker than normal (one-sided weakness indicates damage to the opposite side of the brain; you are testing the motor cortex situated in the frontal lobes but whose motor fibres decuss in the brainstem) or there may be severe weakness.
- Second, assess if the limbs move spontaneously or with painful stimuli or not at all. Score limbs separately if they are different.

Some examples:

- Normal power in arms moving spontaneously scores with two dots; one alongside the normal power box and one alongside the spontaneous box. Normal power in legs moving spontaneously scores two more dots; one alongside the normal power box and one alongside the spontaneous box.
- Normal spontaneous movement in arms (two dots; one alongside the normal power box and one alongside the spontaneous box) but mild weakness with spontaneous movements in the legs (two dots; one alongside the mild weakness box and one alongside the spontaneous box).
- Normal spontaneous movement in right (R) arm (an R alongside the normal power box and an R alongside the spontaneous box) and severe weakness in the left (L) arm responding to painful stimuli only (an L alongside severe weakness and an L alongside painful stimuli).

Pupil size and reaction

The occulomotor cranial nerve (CN III, mixed nerve) arises in the midbrain in the brainstem and is responsible for pupil constriction (Tortora & Grabowski 2003). Pupils in young children tend to be larger and more responsive to light (May 2001).

In a slightly darkened room:

- Observe the size and shape and equality of the pupils; compare the size of the pupil to that in the neurological observation chart (usually measured in millimetres) and document the size of the pupils.
- Cover one of the child's eyes and shine a light into the other; the pupil should constrict briskly (known as a direct light response); withdrawal of light should result in immediate dilation. Now repeat with the other eye. Document as brisk, sluggish or no reaction.
- Observe one pupil and shine the light again into the other pupil; the observed pupil should also constrict (known as consensual response – fibres cross over in the optic chiasma), then repeat with the other eye (Bickley 2003). Document any anomalies in the comments section.

Abnormalities (May 2001):

- Conditions causing pressure on the oculomotor nerve including cerebral oedema or lesions will cause a sluggish papillary response.
- Conditions causing extreme pressure on the oculomotor nerve including brain herniation will result in fixed dilated pupils.
- A one-sided fixed dilated pupil indicates a condition putting extreme pressure on one side of the brain, e.g. herniation (pressure on the nerve reduces the constrictor effect on the pupil and the dilator effects of sympathetic nerves take over).
- With severe hypoxia or infarction, pupils may be in a mid position and non-reactive (neither sympathetic nor parasympathetic innervation is occurring).
- Atropine-like drugs cause pupil dilation, so care with interpretation is required.
- Opioid-type drugs cause pupil constriction, so care with interpretation is required.
- The pons in the brainstem controls many motor pathways and if damaged may result in very small pinpoint non-reactive pupils.

Note that:

- Eyes must be able to open: if the child has peri-orbital oedema, is chemically paralysed or has oculomotor (CN III) nerve damage, he/she cannot open eyes.
- Children may 'play games' and not open or close eyes for you. It may be better to observe them in between observations.
- The frightened child may not co-operate with you and gentle persuasion is needed; involve the family.
- Facial grimace cannot be expressed in the paralysed patient.
- Motor responses originate from the motor cortex and corticospinal/pyramidal tracts and cannot be elicited in the paralysed child.
- Cannulation or trauma may affect limb mobility.

- Normally pupils are round; oval or irregular shapes may indicate brain damage (Shah 1999).

Vital signs

- Respirations: direct pressure on the respiratory centre in the brain stem causes an irregular respiratory rate/apnoea.
- Pulse: in response to hypoxia from raised intracranial pressure, the pulse may increase early to try to increase blood flow to the brain but will then slow, become weak and stop if pressure is not relieved.
- Blood pressure: may be relatively stable with a small rise in ICP but will rise to try to get blood to the brain with higher ICP.
- Cushing's response: as the ICP further increases, the BP rises, the pulse falls and respiratory pattern alters, then the BP will drop, with ensuing death (Vernon-Levett 2001).
- Temperature: temperature regulation is lost when there is pressure on the hypothalamus.

Significant events box

Neurological observations need to be interpreted within the clinical context and this includes any particular events occurring for the child. Note in this section any of the following:

- any medication affecting the conscious level of the patient, e.g. benzodiazepines;
- any seizures;
- any procedures, e.g. theatre, MRI.

DETERMINING MENTAL STATUS BY AVPU
(Basic skill)

Mental status can be determined by the acronym AVPU:

> A = Alert
> V = Responds to voice (as above)
> P = Responds to pain (as above)
> U = Unresponsive to any stimuli

The above method of stimulating a response can be used to determine a quick neurological status (Resuscitation Council (UK) 2004). The P corresponds to a GCS of 8 (Stack & Dobbs

2004). Best practice recommends intubation and ventilation at this score (NICE 2003).

SEIZURES
(Basic skill)

Seizures are brief malfunctions of the brain's electrical system, resulting from cortical neuronal damage, and produce disturbances in behaviour, sensation or motor function (Vernon-Levett 2001). When a child has a seizure, the priority is to keep the child safe and not to restrain him or her. Place in the recovery position, stay with the child and ask for medical assistance for prolonged seizures, any injury that occurs or if respiratory function is abnormal. Further, assess for:

- if there was, and what form, an aura takes;
- activity prior to seizure;
- the length of time of the seizure – time of onset and duration;
- description of the seizure (see Table 7.1);
- time taken to recover post-ictally, changes in behaviour, changes in neurological assessment, duration of sleeping, any confusion.

Table 7.1 Seizure activity (Vernon-Levett 2001).

Seizure	Assessment
Tonic Autonomic overactivity	• Body stiffening • The child may cry out (air is pushed out through vocal cords) • The child may fall • Salivation • Dilated pupils • Tachycardia • Increased blood pressure • May have brief apnoeic episodes
Clonic	• Rhythmical jerking (motor system becomes involved) • One or both sides of the body affected • May include eyes, face, trunk as well as limbs

Table 7.1 Continued.

Seizure	Assessment
Tonic-clonic (major) Also known as grand mal	• The child stiffens and jerks (as above) • The child usually falls • Usually the stiffening occurs first for about $^1/_2$ minute then the jerking for 1–2 minutes
Myoclonic	• Brief, sudden sharp jerking of the limbs • More often upper limbs • May occur more frequently first thing in the morning or at night • May be focal or generalised
Atonic drops	• All muscle stiffness is suddenly lost • The child falls (loss of muscle tone) • If only brief, the knees may give way but child recovers before falling • Injury may occur with falling
Absence Also known as petit mal	• Child appears to be 'in another world' • Usually lasts 5–10 seconds • Sometimes the eyelids blink • If walking the body may sag but usually does not fall • May occur very frequently throughout the day
Complex partial	• Loss of consciousness (reticular formation system involved) • The child may have automatisms – movements that appear strange, e.g. licking lips, swallowing, picking, chewing (Campbell & McIntosh 1998)
Simple partial	• The child can be fully aware • The child may sense strange sensations, e.g. funny feelings in the gut • There may be automatisms; may be clonic jerking
Status epilepticus The abnormal electrical activity involves all areas of the brain, with subsequent potential neuronal death	• Prolonged or recurrent tonic-clonic seizures lasting for 30 minutes or more • **Is a medical emergency** • Respiratory and cardiovascular compromise/ collapse

INTRACRANIAL PRESSURE (ICP)

Normal ICP in adults is 0–15 mm Hg and in infants 0–8 mmHg (James 1989). ICP can be raised due to:

- space-occupying lesion – haematoma or tumour
- cerebral oedema
- hydrocephalus

Because the sutures in an infant's cranium are not completely fused and with open fontanelles, head circumference may expand to accommodate a small increase in ICP.

Look for signs of raised ICP (basic skill):

- Drowsiness: pressure on the reticular activating system will alter the level of consciousness, causing drowsiness and leading to coma and death if the pressure is not reduced.
- Irritability and high-pitched cry: pressure on the reticular activating system can also have an impact on the behaviour of the child and infant.
- Headache: the large arteries (including the middle meningeal arteries), venous sinuses and the dura at the base of the brain are all sensitive to pain due to a high sensory provision and so any pressure or changes to these will cause a headache.
- Vomiting: the vagal motor centres in the brainstem (pons) are associated with vomiting so any pressure on the brain stem may cause vomiting.
- Slow gastro-intestinal motility and gastric emptying.
- Papilloedema: the subdural and subarachnoid spaces will reflect the increased pressure and these spaces are closely associated with the optic nerve (CN II) which becomes oedematous; the optic disc becomes blurred and the retinal veins swell, leading to a decreased visual acuity and then blindness (Hickey 2003).
- Setting sun sign: the iris is directed downward and you can see the sclera above it.
- Bulging fontanelle: an increase in pressure inside the skull will cause the fontanelle to bulge (Stack & Dobbs 2004).
- Decreased blood pressure and heart rate are late signs.

Check that (basic skill):

- The head of the bed is elevated to 15–30°.
- The head is in a neutral midline position.
- The environment is comfortable; not too hot or cold, is quiet and still with light at a minimum.
- Any fever is aggressively managed.
- Any pain is managed.
- Any seizures are managed.
- Airways are maintained and any secretions removed.
- Movement is reduced; sedation should be used as necessary, with extra used for noxious procedures.
- Fluid status and cardiovascular assessment is undertaken frequently (see Chapters 4 and 10).
- Nutrition is commenced as soon as possible (see Chapter 9).
- Care is performed as necessary and one activity at a time to prevent the accumulative effect of clustering care.

ICP monitoring
(Advanced skill)

Following cranial surgery, head trauma, metabolic derangement or a hypoxic-ischaemic insult, an ICP monitor may be placed to measure the intracranial pressure so that trends or changes are managed early (May 2001). Catheters may be placed in the epidural or subarachnoid spaces but more commonly in the brain tissue or lateral ventricle (Rogers 1996). Ventricular catheterisation has the added advantage of being able to drain cerebrospinal fluid if necessary (see below).

Look for:

- signs of infection at the site (rare) (Adelson *et al.* 2003);
- any bleeding at the site;
- any tension on the catheter (Hazinski 1992).

The catheter is connected to a transducer (see Chapter 5) for waveform and numerical monitoring on a monitor screen. Transducer systems may be:

- fluid-filled (but no flushing) and require regular zeroing (according to local protocol). The transducer's anatomic reference point is usually at the middle ear (see Figure 7.3, below) and levelling will be required whenever the patient's position is changed;

- fibreoptic, requiring calibrating and zeroing prior to insertion and after any disconnection (e.g. Codman system). The reference pressure point is in the tip of the catheter so there is no re-levelling requirement with position changes of the patient.

Check the waveform:

- its resemblance to the arterial waveform (see Chapter 5), albeit with different amplitudes;
- its synchronicity with arterial pulsation;
- whether respiratory pattern fluctuations are seen (reflecting the transmission of the intrapleural pressure to the cranium) (Rogers 1996);
- there may be normal transient rises with coughing. Figure 7.2 shows an example of the three intracranial waveforms, which are described below.

Waveforms identified by Lundberg (1960) include:

(1) *Plateau or A waves*. From normal or already slightly elevated pressures there is a slow rise to high pressures, often over 50 mmHg (Hickey 2003). Without management, these high pressures may persist for up to 20 minutes prior to falling. They represent a loss of cerebral autoregulation and result

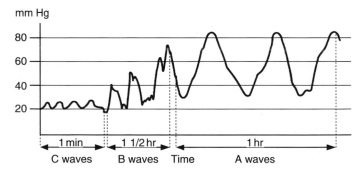

Fig. 7.2 Intracranial pressure waveforms.

in brain hypoperfusion due to hypoxia, hypercapnoea or oedema, and are considered an ominous event. Further management of raised ICP is required.

(2) *B waves*. These are more frequent recordings. They represent rhythmic waves that may fluctuate with respirations, have pointed peaks and range from 20–50 mmHg. These waves may indicate developing coma (Hazinski 1992) and are associated with inadequate respiratory status (Hickey 2003). Neurological assessment and management may need reviewing.

(3) *C waves*. These are smaller low-amplitude waves that can occur up to eight times per minute, with no variance with respirations and unclear clinical significance.

As well as hourly recordings, document all spiking of ICP measurements and undertake associated neurological examination (as above).

CEREBRAL PERFUSION PRESSURE (CPP)
(Advanced skill)

ICP catheters are often inserted so that cerebral perfusion pressure (CPP) can be measured to ensure adequate perfusion (and therefore oxygen and glucose) to the brain to meet its metabolic needs. CPP requires a mean arterial pressure (MAP) reading, usually supplied by an invasive arterial catheter attached to a transducer (see Chapter 5).

$$CPP = MAP - ICP$$

Normal CPP in children is unknown but thought to be 40–60 mmHg (Palmer 2000). There appears to be a greater mortality with CPPs < 40 mmHg (Adelson *et al* 2003). As ICP increases towards the MAP level, blood flow to the brain becomes less and less, with death occurring when there is no blood flow.

(Write here your clinical unit's guidelines for CPP levels:)

In managing CPP, check that:

- assessments are undertaken frequently for signs of raised ICP (see above);

- the patient's ventilation and oxygenation status is as normal as possible (see Chapters 2 and 3);
- any external ventricular drainage system is functioning (see below).

Record CPP hourly and any abnormal fluctuations in between.

EXTERNAL VENTRICULAR DRAINS (EVD)

(Advanced skill)

Catheters may be inserted into the ventricle for drainage of cerebrospinal fluid (CSF) and are often used in conjunction with ICP monitoring (see above). CSF may need to be drained if there is excess (e.g. in hydrocephalus) or to reduce a raised ICP (Hazinski 1992).

Check that:

- An IV stand is placed next to the head of the bed and a tape measure is taped to the pole, with the zero at the patient's anatomical reference point – the interventricular foramen (foramen of Monro). This is at:
  - o the middle ear/external auditory canal in older children;
  - o the mid-point between the ear and the corner of the eye in infants (Terry & Nisbet 1991).

See Fig. 7.3 for middle ear anatomical reference points for the child and infant.

- The drainage drip chamber is levelled at the prescribed level (usually 10–15 cm H_2O) above the anatomical reference point so that when ICP rises, CSF drains (the higher the level, the higher the ICP will have to be for CSF to drain) (Cummings 1992).
- Accuracy of levelling is ensured by using a spirit level, laser tool or length of tubing joined and filled with coloured fluid (see Chapter 5) (Bisnaire & Robinson 1997).
- The child is relatively settled with head of bed elevated (discuss with neurosurgeon), but if the child raises his or her head above the level of the drip chamber, CSF will drain by gravity, which may cause ventricular collapse.

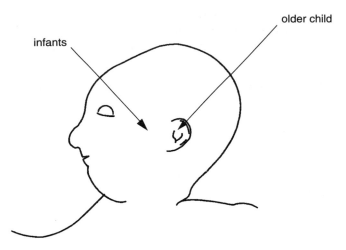

Fig. 7.3 Middle ear anatomical reference points for the child and infant.

- The system is closed temporarily (turn off clamp closest to the patient) when repositioning the child and the anatomical reference point/drip chamber is re-levelled.
- All clamps between the drip chamber and catheter are open.
- All connections are secure.
- The tubing is not kinked or twisted.
- All tubing is clearly labelled.
- Any pain is assessed and managed (see Chapter 14).
- Monitor and document CSF colour and volume losses hourly.
- If CSF losses cease abruptly, obstruction from blood or tissue may have occurred; check medical orders for flushing the line (usually a medical role).
- Neurological assessment is undertaken frequently (hourly).
- Drainage bags are changed when three-quarters full, using a sterile technique (Gibson 1995).
- Signs of infection and bleeding, although rare (Rogers 1996), are observed for.

- Samples are taken for culture as per local policy:
  - an aseptic technique is used;
  - isolate the tap closest to the patient and turn it off to patient for a few minutes to allow buildup of fluid;
  - remove cap in the meantime and clean well with alcohol, waiting at least a full minute for it to dry;
  - open the tap to air below the level of the catheter and allow 1–2 ml of CSF to drip into a sterile pot held under the tap (do not aspirate);
  - turn the tap off to air and replace cap with new one.
- The catheter is removed in a timely manner:
  - medical orders have been given;
  - sutures are removed if used;
  - the catheter is slowly but continually pulled for removal;
  - the catheter is intact when removed;
  - sutures are placed (by medical staff) if required;
  - the wound is dressed and inspected frequently for leakage of CSF or bleeding;
  - neurological assessment is undertaken frequently following catheter removal (Cummings 1992).

JUGULAR VENOUS BULB MONITORING
(Advanced skill)

This is a technique for measuring adequate global perfusion and hence oxygen consumption of the brain. A fibre-optic catheter is passed into the jugular vein in a retrograde fashion towards the jugular venous bulb at the base of the skull where normal jugular venous bulb oxygen saturations (SjO_2) are 65–70%. If there is a reduced blood flow or oxygen delivery to the brain, there will be a fall in the venous saturation. Venous saturations of 40% indicate ischaemia (Stack & Dobbs 2004). An increase in SjO_2 may indicate an increase in cerebral blood flow or tissue necrosis.

Check SjO_2 monitoring for:

- light intensity;
- alarm settings: the practitioner needs to decide at what point he/she wants to know the reading has changed, and set the alarms accordingly;

- for an adequate trace on the screen;
- that the clinical condition correlates with the SjO_2 results.

Check the patient for:

- normal haemoglobin;
- adequate arterial oxygenation and ventilation;
- cannulation site complications of infection and bleeding (see Chapter 14).

CEREBRAL FUNCTION ANALYSIS MONITORING (CFAM)
(Advanced skill)

An electroencephalogram (EEG) is a recording of the electrical activity of the brain and can be obtained using the standard 19-electrode method; however, this is time-consuming and impractical and requires expert interpretation. Continuous bedside monitoring is available in the form of cerebral function analysis monitoring (CFAM).

Two symmetrical pairs of scalp electrodes are applied. They are applied in the F3/P3 and F4/P4 positions, i.e. in the middle of the left and right parietal and frontal cranial bones (Murdoch-Eaton *et al.* 2001). However, check manufacturer's instructions for positioning.

CFAM:

- provides detailed information on background electrical activity; amplitude and frequencies and symmetry:
  o with decreased cerebral blood flow, EEG rhythms are reduced in both amplitude and frequency;
  o following an hypoxic-ischaemic injury, EEG rhythms can be examined for return of cognitive function;
  o with a barbiturate coma, EEG rhythms can be interpreted for suppression of electrical activity (Vernon-Levett 2001).
- provides information on added electrical activities such as seizures, and brief or prolonged electrical activity (Murdoch-Eaton *et al.* 2001).

Check that:

- the electrodes are well secured to the scalp;
- all connections are secure;

- the monitor is calibrated as per manufacturer's instructions;
- documentation is in line with local policy.

TRAIN-OF-FOUR (TOF) TESTING
(Advanced skill)

Train-of-four (TOF) testing is a technique used to assess the level of neuromuscular blockade (NMB) when the patient has had neuromuscular blocking agents administered. Optimising the drug therapy and reducing complications (muscular weakness, inability to wean from ventilation) can be achieved by monitoring the level of blockade. However, in adults no differences in drug doses or duration of paralysis were found when TOF testing was used compared to clinical assessment (Baumann *et al.* 2004).

Two cutaneous paediatric ECG electrodes are placed 5–10 cm apart along the nerve. When a small electrical stimulus is applied to the nerve with an intact neuromuscular junction, the muscle supplied by the nerve will contract. The effect of the NMB is evaluated by the decrease in this muscle activity (Henneman *et al.* 1995). Table 7.2 shows the different nerves that can be used.

Check:

- the electrodes are well sealed on the skin and correctly placed;
- all connections are secure;
- where possible nerve stimulation is carried out prior to neuromuscular blockade to establish a baseline or threshold of the

Table 7.2 Nerves that can be used in train-of-four testing.

Nerve	Location	Muscle	Effect
Distal ulnar	At the wrist in line with the little finger	Ulnar nerve- adductor pollicis	Thumb will adduct
Facial	Slightly inferior and lateral to the eye	Orbicularis occuli	Eyelid twitch
Sural	Below and lateral to the medial malleolus of the ankle	Flexor hallucis brevis	Plantar flexion (curling up) of the big toe

amount of milliamps required to elicit a single twitch, then double this as the starting point for use in evaluating neuro-muscular blockade (Henneman *et al.* 1995);
- the peripheral nerve stimulator is fully charged;
- the distal electrode is connected to the negative terminal (may be black);
- the proximal electrode is connected to the positive terminal (may be red);
- TOF delivers four stimuli (2 Hz) at 0.5 second apart;
- the level of paralysis requirement with medical staff;
- and feel for twitches by placing the patient's hand palm-up, gently abducting the thumb and resting fingertips on it. Visualise the twitches as well as thumb adduction and plantar flexion of the big toe;
- and document stimulus level and number of twitches;
- and repeat testing (e.g. every 15–30 minutes) until level of neuromuscular blockade required is attained, and then 4–8 hourly, depending on local policy.

Table 7.3 shows interpretation of results when the patient has been receiving neuromuscular drug therapy (but not immediately following a bolus).

Table 7.3 Interpretation of results of train-of-four testing. (Data for percentage of receptors blocked came from Organon Inc. (undated) *Train of Four: Peripheral Nerve Stimulation.* Organon Inc, New Jersey.)

Number of twitches	Percentage of receptors blocked	Interpretation
0	100	May be desired for intubation Patient is over-paralysed Decrease dose
1	90	Appropriate level
2	80	Appropriate level
3	75	Inadequate neuromuscular blockade Increase dose
4	0–75	Inadequate neuromuscular blockade May see clinical signs of moving Increase dose

---

Case Study

Joe is a 6-year-old boy who has been knocked off his bicycle whilst on his way to school by a car travelling at 40 miles/hour. At the scene Joe was unconscious with a GCS of 7. No other injuries were obvious. He was intubated and ventilated by the paramedics and taken to the nearest Emergency Department. You undertake his neurological recordings, chart and report a GCS of 3 (Joe has been sedated – noted in the significant events box), pupils both size 5 with sluggish reaction, responds weakly to painful stimuli equally in all limbs, temperature 36.2, blood pressure 90/45, pulse 135, and respirations non-existent above the ventilator. There are no signs of fitting. His ABGs show good oxygenation, normal pH and a low to normal $PaCO_2$ level.

Based on these findings, he is transferred to the MRI scanner where a diagnosis of cerebral oedema is made and he is transferred to theatre for insertion of an intracranial pressure monitor. Upon return to the unit, he is connected to the monitor for ECG, blood pressure and ICP monitoring. His ICP is 35 with waves that resemble B waves. CPP is 20. The catheter does not have a ventricular drainage system and drug therapy is introduced to reduce the increased ICP. You attach a CFAM which shows decreased amplitude and frequency of waves.

SUMMARY

Assessing and monitoring the neurological status of all sick children enables baseline recordings and early detection of clinical status. However, there can be a subjective nature to examination and therefore staff handing over must establish inter-observer reliability. It is also in the child's best interests to work closely with parents/carers to establish what is normal for that child. The use of technological monitoring can assist clinical decision-making, but appropriate health and safety training must be undertaken.

REFERENCES

Adelson, P.D., Bratton, S.L., Carney, N.A., *et al.* (2003) Guidelines for the acute medical management of severe traumatic brain injury in infants, children and adolescents. *Pediatric Critical Care Medicine*, **4** (3) (Suppl.).

Baumann, M.H., McAlpin, B.W., Brown, K., *et al.* (2004) A prospective randomized comparison of train-of-four monitoring and clinical assessment during continuous ICU cisatracurium paralysis. *Chest*, **126**, 1267–1273.

Bickley, L.S. (2003) *Bates Guide to Physical Examination and History Taking*, 8th edn. Lippincott, Williams and Wilkins, Philadelphia, Chapter 16.

Bisnaire, D. & Robinson, L. (1997) Accuracy of levelling intraventricular collection drainage systems. *Journal of Neuroscience Nursing*, **29** (1), 261–268.

Campbell, A.G.M. & McIntosh, N. (1998) *Forfar and Arneil's Textbook of Pediatrics*, 5th edn. Churchill Livingston, New York.

Cummings, R. (1992) Understanding external ventricular drainage. *Journal of Neuroscience Nursing*, **24** (2), 84–87.

Gibson, I. (1995) Making sense of external ventricular drainage. *Nursing Times*, **91** (23), 34–35.

Gill, D. & O'Brien, N. (2002) *Paediatric Clinical Examination Made Easy*, 4th edn. Churchill Livingston, Edinburgh.

Hazinski, M.F. (1992) *Nursing Care of the Critically Ill Child*, 2nd edn. Mosby, St Louis.

Henneman, E.A., Bellamy, P. & Togashi, C. (1995) Peripheral nerve stimulators in the critical care setting: a policy for monitoring neuromuscular blockade. *Critical Care Nurse*, June, 82–88.

Hickey, J.V. (2003) *The Clinical Practice of Neurological and Neurosurgical Nursing*, 5th edn. Lippincott, New York.

Lundberg, N. (1960) Continuous recording and control of ventricular fluid pressure in neurosurgical practice. *Acta Psychiatrica et Neurologica Scandiavia*, **36** (149), 1–193.

May, L. (2001) *Paediatric Neuro-surgery; A Handbook for the Multidisciplinary Team*. Hurr, London.

Monaghan, A. (2005) Detecting and managing deterioration in children. *Paediatric Nursing*, **17** (1), 32–35.

Murdoch-Eaton, D., Darowski, M. & Livingston, J. (2001) Cerebral function monitoring in paediatric intensive care: useful features for predicting outcome. *Developmental Medicine and Child Neurology*, **43**, 91–96.

National Institute for Clinical Excellence (2003) *Triage, Assessment, Investigation and Early Management of Head Injuries in Infants, Children and Adults: Clinical Guideline 4*. NICE, London.

Palmer, J. (2000) Management of raised intracranial pressure in children. *Intensive and Critical Care Nursing*, **16**, 319–327.

Resuscitation Council (UK) (2004) *European Paediatric Life Support Course Provider Manual*. Resuscitation Council (UK), London.

Rogers, M. (ed) (1996) *Textbook of Pediatric Intensive Care*, 3rd edn. Williams and Wilkins, Baltimore.

Shah, S. (1999) Neurological assessment. *Nursing Standard*, **13** (22), 49–54.

Stack, C. & Dobbs, P. (2004) *Essentials of Paediatric Intensive Care*. GMM, London.

Terry, D. & Nisbet, K. (1991) Nursing care of the child with external ventricular drainage. *Journal of Neuroscience Nursing*, **23** (6), 347–353.

Tortora, G.J. & Grabowski, S.R. (2003) *Principles of Anatomy and Physiology*, 10th edn. John Wiley, New York.

Vernon-Levett, P. (2001) Intracranial dynamics. In: Curley, M.A.Q and Moloney-Harmon, P.A. eds. *Critical Care Nursing of Infants and Children* (2nd ed). W.B. Saunders Company, Philadelphia

Warren, A. (2000) Paediatric coma scoring researched and benchmarked. *Paediatric Nursing*, **12** (3), 14–18.

The Gastro-intestinal System and Abdomen

8

INTRODUCTION

Gastro-intestinal (GI) assessment in infants and children is critical in evaluating growth and development, as well as the pathophysiological impact of illness. Examination of the abdomen provides information about the internal organs and nutrition/feeding. When examining the child, the health care practitioner will choose a range of techniques depending on the clinical presentation. The aim of this chapter is to understand the principles of gastro-intestinal system assessment and monitoring for different age groups.

LEARNING OBJECTIVES

By the end of this chapter the reader will be able to:

❏ Appreciate the importance of taking a history.
❏ Outline the steps of a comprehensive assessment.
❏ Understand the GI system assessment of vomiting and bleeding.

HISTORY

Reviewing this system should include asking about:

- ability to suck or eat, and appetite;
- palate anomalies;
- feeding abnormalities, food allergies and intolerances;
- feeding history including type, frequency and amount of intake, who feeds the child, who prepares food; breast fed or bottle fed;
- regurgitation/vomiting – neonates do not develop full muscle tone of the lower oesophageal sphincter until 1 month of age

so regurgitation of feeds is normal (Engel 1997) – or any gastro-oesophageal reflux;

- bowel pattern including constipation and diarrhoea or rectal bleeding;
- weight loss or gain outwith normal;
- recent trauma/infection;
- underlying chronic illnesses or disease;
- abdominal pain including frequency, intensity, type and location;
- review of medications and their effect on the GI system.

PHYSICAL EXAMINATION
Head and neck
(See Chapter 11)

- Assess for jaundice: examine the sclera, tongue and conjunctiva.
- Examine the mouth for:
  - pale mucous membranes indicating anaemia;
  - halitosis, ulcers (known as apthous ulcers) and sores.

Abdomen
Visceral pain is the most common type of pain in children, e.g. colicky pain of the intestine or appendicitis. The pain can be easily referred and the child will be restless. Parietal pain is well localised and the child lies still to prevent movement. Rebound tenderness testing is not always recommended in children (Bagnell 1997) as careful palpation will provide adequate information. Examine all quadrants of the abdomen as shown in Fig. 8.1 from the patient's right side if possible.

Ensure that your hands are warm and nails are short. Bowel sounds may be affected by handling of the abdomen and therefore the techniques of examination are undertaken in the order detailed below (Engel 1997):

Inspection
(Basic skill)
- Expose entire abdomen and look at the contour directly and from an angle, looking for any bulges or visible organs, e.g.

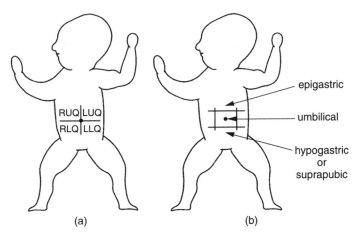

Fig. 8.1a,b The abdominal areas (*RUQ* right upper quadrant; *LUQ* left upper quadrant; *RLQ* right lower quadrant; *LLQ* left lower quadrant).

loops of bowel, any rashes, scars or lesions, or peristalsis; the umbilicus for inflammation, contour or herniation; the inguinal area for herniation (especially in male infants) (Gill & O'Brien 2002).
- The abdomen is normally flat or slightly rounded when supine, but when standing, it is normal to have a pot belly until puberty, related to the immature curvature of the spine.

Auscultation
(Basic skill)
- Listen with the diaphragm in the right lower quadrant (RLQ) for gurgles, clicks or growls; you may want to listen in all four quadrants.
- Listen for a minimum of 5 minutes before deciding there are no bowel sounds. Note that the presence or absence of bowel sounds does not accurately reflect the gut's ability to absorb feeds.

Percussion
(Advanced skill)

For technique see Chapter 1. Check for dullness over organs and masses, e.g. liver, and tympany over air, e.g. stomach or gas in the bowel. Infants may have more tympanic sounds as they tend to swallow air (Szilagyi 2003).

Palpation
(Basic skill)

- Feel the abdomen to confirm visible, auscultatory or percussion findings and any abnormally large organs or masses, areas of tenderness, guarding and fullness (Bagnell 1997).
- Place hands on abdomen and apply light pressure with fingertips, checking for tenderness, before pushing a little deeper throughout the entire abdomen. If you are able to get the child's co-operation in 'puffing out' and 'sucking in' the stomach, the degree of tenderness may be determined prior to deep palpation (Engel 1997).
- Children and infants need to be relaxed, and distraction techniques and patience are required.
  - It may be helpful to flex the child's head or hips, perhaps using pillows (Engel 1997). It is easy to hold the infant's legs in a flexed position with one hand (Szilagyi 2003).
  - A child crawling or sitting up may be more co-operative (Gill & O'Brien 2002).
  - Asking the child to put his or her hand over yours when palpating may decrease 'ticklishness' (Engel 1997).

Checking for ascites
(Basic skill)

Check for ascites by noting the following:

- a distended abdomen;
- free fluid in the abdomen;
- an umbilicus turning outward;
- oedematous skin;
- swollen scrotum or vulva;
- flanks (the area between the ribs and iliac crest) becoming more solid and bulging;

- shifting dullness (advanced skill):
  - when the patient is supine, the flanks will give a dull percussion note;
  - turn the child onto his or her side;
  - wait for up to a minute to allow the fluid to settle (Gill & O'Brien 2002);
  - on percussion, the upper flank will produce a tympanic note from the gas-filled bowel (the fluid has sunk with gravity).

Spleen
(Advanced skill)

Percussion

- The percussion technique is outlined in Chapter 1.
- Percuss in the left upper quadrant (LUQ) in the anterior axilla line just below the costal margin, then downwards towards the iliac fossa, then medially towards the umbilicus and then laterally to the mid-axilla line.
- A dull percussion note will be found over the organ; this is known as a positive splenic percussion sign.
- A positive splenic percussion sign can suggest a splenomegaly (Bickley 2003).
- The spleen may normally be found 1–2 cm below the costal margin (Gill & O'Brien 2002).

Palpation

- Place your left hand under the patient's left lower rib cage and gently pull it forward.
- Place the fingertips of the right hand below the umbilicus and gently press into the abdomen; release, and using the technique of press/release, slowly move towards the spleen.
- Respiration will push the spleen forward so note if and where the splenic tip comes to meet the fingertips.
- Note the size of the spleen in centimetres below the costal margin.
- Palpation can confirm a splenomegaly but may miss those enlarged spleens that do not descend below the costal margin.

Liver
(Advanced skill)

Palpation
- Stand on the child's right side.
- For an infant, it may be easier to use the tip of the right thumb.
- For a child, use fingers.
- Begin well down in the right lower quadrant (RLQ) of the abdomen and press inward and upward, then release. Using this technique, move slowly up toward the liver.
- It is helpful if the patient can take a large breath, but in children this co-operation is not always available.
- There may be a sense of resistance during progression up the abdomen.
- The liver edge can normally be found (Campbell & McIntosh 1998):
  - above the right costal margin (RCM) in young people and adults;
  - at 1 cm below the costal margin in 4- to 5-year-old children;
  - at 2 cm below the costal margin in 1-year-old children;
  - at 3 cm below the costal margin in infants.
- Always watch the child closely for signs of distress and liver tenderness.
- Lung hyperinflation will push the liver down, giving an impression of hepatomegaly; liver size may be better determined by percussion.

Percussion
This technique can be used to confirm palpation findings or further determine liver size if the liver edge is soft and it is difficult to find the margin. For details on percussion technique, see Chapter 1.

- Percuss along the midclavicular line from well down in the right lower quadrant (RLQ) of the abdomen, moving towards the thorax, noting when the sound becomes dull; this will be the liver edge.

- Estimate the number of centimetres below the costal margin the liver edge is.

To determine the vertical span of the liver:

- Percuss along the midclavicular line from the right upper lung lobe, moving down towards the abdomen, noting when the sound becomes dull; this will be the upper liver edge.
- Using a ruler, measure the difference between the upper and lower edges of the liver. Table 8.1 shows normal liver span values for different ages (Gill & O'Brien 2002; Bickley 2003).

The scratch test

This technique can be used to determine the lower border of the liver, although some practitioners have not found this technique useful in children (Gill & O'Brien 2002).

- Identify the right midclavicular line and place the diaphragm of the stethoscope just above the right costal margin.
- *Lightly* scratch the child's skin with a fingernail along the midclavicular line, moving from below the level of the umbilicus towards the stethoscope.
- The scratching sound changes as it meets the liver edge and passes through the liver to the stethoscope (Bickley 2003).
- Estimate the number of centimetres below the costal margin the liver edge is.

Bladder

(Advanced skill)

In the neonate and infant, the bladder is an abdominal organ rather than a pelvic organ (MacGregor 2001).

Table 8.1 Normal liver span values.

Age	Liver span (cm)
Infant	2–3 (mean)
Toddler	3–4 (mean)
School age	4–5 (mean)
6 years to adolescence	6–12 (range)

- A full bladder may be seen in the hypogastric area.
- A full bladder will have a dull percussion note (see Chapter 1 for technique).
- Use the fingertips to palpate the bladder.

Genitalia
(Advanced)
Although not strictly part of the gastro-intestinal system, it may be pertinent to include this aspect of examination. *Examination of the genitalia should only be undertaken within the health care practitioner's scope of practice. Also, some aspects of examination may be appropriate for some practices and other practices may not warrant any aspect of the examination at all. It may be that health care professionals observe some aspects during routine hygiene cares. If examination is required, consider carefully whether or not a chaperone is required, e.g. another health care professional or a parent, and use legal and professional guidelines.*

Inspection provides as much information as palpation. Ensure your hands are warm. A more detailed guide to childhood sexual development can be found in other literature, e.g. in Tanner (1962). Sexual abuse assessment is not covered in this book.

Male
- Penis
  - Look to see that the urethra opens onto the end of the penis and not underneath (hypospadias) or above (epispadias).
  - Note the size (micropenia is rare) (Gill & O'Brien 2002).
- Scrotum and testes
  - Inspect the foreskin (non-retractable at birth).
  - Look for normal scrotal wrinkling and the presence of testes.
  - Palpate testes for presence and size:
    - place first and second fingers behind the scrotum;
    - using the thumb, palpate downwards from the groin.
  - Note that testes easily retract and the examination may have to be repeated.
  - The child may prefer standing rather than lying down.

○ It may be useful to have the child sit cross-legged and have him blow up a balloon or lift an object to increase intra-abdominal pressure (Bickley 2003).

○ An enlarged scrotum may indicate an inguinal hernia or an hydrocele (common in neonates).

Female
- Inspect the vulva and check for any adhesions or rashes.
- Note the clitoris can be normally enlarged in the neonate, due to the mother's oestrogen levels (Bickley 2003).
- Gently separate the labia and note labia minora, urethra, vagina and hymen for any swelling, inflammation, bleeding or discharge.

Anal area
Inspect the anus, buttocks and thighs for

- a perforate anus in neonates;
- marks or trauma, anal fissures, polyps, tags or haemorrhoids (rare);
- redness, rash, bleeding, faecal staining or infection;
- threadworms.

Rectal examinations are not routinely performed and are only undertaken for diagnostic purposes.

VOMITING
(Basic skill)
Vomiting is relatively common in childhood and the following should be assessed:

- amount;
- frequency and timing;
- contents and consistency (Table 8.2 shows the definition of some terms);
- forceful or passive;
- any relation to specific events, e.g. feeding, stress, high temperature, pain (Bagnell 1997; Gill & O'Brien 2002);
- vomiting in relation to gastric feeding (discussed further in Chapter 9).

Table 8.2 Gastrointestinal terminology.

Term	Definition	Source
Projectile vomit	Vomiting is forceful	May be due to pyloric stenosis (infant) or raised intracranial pressure
Undigested milk/food vomit	Vomiting has occurred before digestion	–
Yellow vomit	May smell acidic	Stomach
Dark green vomit	Bile-stained	Below the ampulla of Vater
Coffee-ground vomit	Old blood in the vomit that has started to be digested	May be a bleed or due to iron tablets
Faecal-smelling vomit	Faecal matter in the vomit	May be indicative of small bowel obstruction (Bagnell 1997)
Meconium	Dark green, smooth and sticky characteristics and is passed within the first 24 hours of life	Normal newborn stool
Soft/liquid faeces	Normal for breast-fed babies	May pass faeces up to 12 times per day
Light yellow/pasty faeces	Normal in formula-fed babies	–
Liquid or watery green faeces	Diarrhoea	Infectious diseases
Firm, hard stool	–	Inadequate diet or fluid intake, obstruction
Frothy or foul-smelling faeces	–	Indicates cystic fibrosis (Engel 1997)
Haematemesis	Bright red vomiting	Bleeding in duodenum above ligament of Trentz
Haematochezia	Bright red blood or maroon-coloured stool from rectum	Colonic source
Malaena	Dark, black, tarry stools (black as a result of bacteria action on Hb)	Bleeding from above ileocaecal valve
Occult blood	Trace amounts of blood in normal-appearing stools	Chronic bleed

Assess the child or infant for signs of dehydration as vomiting can quickly cause dehydration in young children (see Chapter 10).

DIARRHOEA
(Basic skill)
Table 8.2 also outlines some types of stools. Diarrhoea may be acute, chronic or recurrent. Most is acute in children and due to an infection. Check for:

- amount
- frequency
- content and consistency

Assess the child or infant for signs of dehydration as diarrhoea can quickly cause dehydration in young children (see Chapter 10).

GASTRO-INTESTINAL BLEEDING
(Basic skill)
Children are more likely to suffer upper GI bleeding than lower GI bleeding and a stress-associated GI bleed is a major factor affecting morbidity and mortality (Chaibou *et al.* 1998) especially in those who are critically ill, e.g. with sepsis or head injury.

Look for active bleeding, low haemoglobin and hypotension. Table 8.2 shows the definition of various terms associated with the GI tract.

Case Study

Sally is an 18-month-old child who is brought to the walk-in centre with a 2-day history of crying and 'abdominal pain'.

History
Normally good appetite; takes several milk bottles a day as well as three soft food meals.
Daily soft brown stool patterns passed easily with no pain or bleeding.
Now taking milk but eating less; no vomiting.

Continued

No stools for 3 days; some 'straining' reported by mother.
Normal growth and development patterns.
No known family history of constipation.
No recent illnesses.

On examination
Is a little restless but drinking from a cup.
Slightly distended abdomen.
Bowel sounds heard in RLQ.
Draws legs up and cries with light abdominal palpation in all areas. Small, hard lumps found in umbilical area (?faeces).
Liver 1 cm below the costal margin.
No oedema.
Bladder not palpated.
Anus not inflamed; intact.

Refer Sally for ?constipation.

SUMMARY
Examining the GI system is important for the care of the sick infant and child. Depending on the presentation of the child, the health care practitioner will need to decide which techniques are appropriate to use. Vomiting, diarrhoea and abdominal pain can be common complaints of this age group.

REFERENCES
Bagnell, P. (1997) Clinical evaluation of gastrointestinal symptoms in children. In: Goldbloom RB, *Pediatric Clinical Skills*, 2nd edn. Churchill Livingston, Philadelphia.

Bickley, L.S. (2003) *Bates Guide to Physical Examination and History Taking*, 8th edn. Lippincott, Williams and Wilkins, Philadelphia, Chapter 9.

Campbell, A.G.M. & McIntosh, N. (1998) *Forfar and Arneil's Textbook of Pediatrics*, 5th edn. Churchill Livingston, New York.

Chaibou, M., Tucci, M., Dugas, M.A. & Farrell, C.A. (1998) Clinically significant upper gastrointestinal bleeding acquired in a pediatric intensive care unit: a prospective study. *Pediatrics*, **102** (4), Part 1, 933–938.

Engel, J. (1997) *Pediatric Assessment*, 3rd edn. Mosby, St. Louis.

Gill, D. & O'Brien, N. (2002) *Paediatric Clinical Examination Made Easy*, 4th edn. Churchill Livingston, Edinburgh.

MacGregor, J. (2001) *Introduction to the Anatomy and Physiology of Children*. Routlege, London.

Szilagyi, P.G. (2003) Assessing children: infancy through adolescence. In: Bickley, L.S. (ed) *Bates Guide to Physical Examination and History Taking*, 8th edn. Lippincott, Williams and Wilkins, Philadelphia.

Tanner, J.M. (1962) *Growth at Adolescence*, 2nd edn. Blackwell, Oxford.

9 | Nutrition

INTRODUCTION

Children have a high-energy requirement for growth and development with low ability for nutrient storage and a higher metabolic rate than adults, and are therefore at greater risk of malnutrition. Malnutrition has been found in a significant number of hospitalised children in the UK (Cross *et al.* 1995; Hendrikse *et al.* 1997). Patients who are malnourished often have longer hospital stays (Ekvall *et al.* 2005). Early feeding can have a positive impact on morbidity and mortality (Martinez *et al.* 2004). There is little research found on the nursing management of nutrition in sick children.

LEARNING OBJECTIVES

By the end of this chapter the reader will be able to:

❑ Understand the professional responsibility for nutritional assessment.
❑ Learn techniques in nutritional assessment.
❑ Evaluate the impact of illness on nutrition.
❑ Ensure adequate nutrition for children.
❑ Assess safe practices in administration of feeding.

MALNUTRITION

Malnutrition may be defined as:

• undernutrition: insufficient energy and/or nutrients;
• overnutrition: excess of nutrients.

(BAPEN 2005)

Malnutrition can be caused by:

* overeating: leading to obesity;
* starvation: there is normal *use* of nutrients, just not enough of them; the body rations energy for survival and malnutrition can take days or weeks;
* the metabolic response to stress, e.g. critical illness or trauma: nutrients are unable to be used normally due to the disruption to homeostasis and metabolic activity (Gaw *et al.* 1999).

The metabolic response to stress occurs in three phases (Thomas 1994):

(1) Ebb – lasts for a few hours during which time there is a reduction of energy expenditure as the body rations the use of energy available.
(2) Flow (catabolism) – during this time there is:
    * a further increased basal metabolic rate (BMR);
    * an increase in normal resting energy expenditure (REE; energy that is used for normal metabolic processes in the body);
    * increased gluconeogenesis, glycogenolysis, hyperglycaemia and insulin resistance;
    * protein loss (causing a negative nitrogen balance);
    * lipolysis.

    These biochemical changes are facilitated by cortisol, glucagons and catecholamines that act to save the patient in the short term but have severe consequences (Gaw *et al.* 1999).
(3) Anabolic – during this time, energy and nutrients are starting to be used efficiently as the cause of the stress has been successfully managed.

NUTRITIONAL TRIGGER ASSESSMENT

Government and professional directives (NHS Modernisation Agency 2003; DH 2004a,b; RCN 2006) advise that all children have an initial and then ongoing nutritional assessment; and that all children have a feeding plan and referral when required, e.g. breastfeeding support, health visitor, dietician or paediatrician. NICE (2006) also directs health care professionals to assess their patients' nutritional status.

All equipment must be accurate and adequately maintained, e.g. calibrated scales on an even firm surface. Measurements must be undertaken as accurately and precisely as possible and plotted on growth charts (Ekvall *et al.* 2005). Table 9.1 outlines the process for accurately plotting measurements on the growth charts according to decimal age (basic skill). The Child Growth

Table 9.1 Plotting growth measurements according to decimal age.

To determine decimal age

Use the appropriate gender growth chart and use the decimal year calculation chart

(1) Note the child's date of birth
  • with the year of birth: note the last two figures
  • with the day and month of date of birth: go to the decimal year calculation chart and identify the figure along from the month of birth and down from the date of birth
  • write down the last two figures from the year of birth and the resultant day/month calculation from the chart in the following manner: YY.decimal year calculation figure
(2) Note the date of the recorded measurement and determine a decimalised figure in the same manner as date of birth
(3) Subtract the decimalised child's date of birth from the decimalised measurement date; this gives the decimal age
(4) The measurement should be plotted on the growth chart according to this age

An example: a 3-year-old girl whose date of birth is 26.05.03 and the growth measurements were taken on 26.06.06

(1) Date of birth
  • year of birth: 03
  • day/month calculation from the decimal year calculation chart: 397
  • a final figure of 03.397
(2) Date of recorded measurements
  • year of recorded measurement: 06
  • day/month calculation from the decimal year calculation chart: 482
  • a final figure of 06.482
(3) Subtract date of birth from date of measurement
  • 06.482 minus 03.397 = decimal age of 3.085 or 3.1 years
(4) The measurements should be plotted against the age of 3.1 years

---

Foundation has produced Boys and Girls Four-in-One Growth Charts (Child Growth Foundation 1996a,b). If weight falls more than two centiles over 6 months (for children less than 2 years old) or over 12 months (for children over 2 years) and was not planned, malnutrition should be suspected (RCN 2006).

Weight

(Basic skill)

Although there are variables for normal growth and sex, Table 9.2 shows the average weights for children in the United Kingdom based on the 50th centiles (Cole 1994; Freeman *et al.* 1995; Chinn 1996; Great Ormond Street Hospital for Children NHS Trust 2000).

With appropriate privacy and dignity, children under 3 years should be weighed naked and those over 3 years with very minimal clothing. Ensure the child is placed centrally on the scales and is still at the time of reading the measurement (RCN

Table 9.2 Average weights (in kilogrammes) of babies and children according to age and gender. (Adapted from Great Ormond Street Hospital for Children NHS Trust (2000) *Nutritional Requirements for Children in Health and Disease.*)

Age	Male	Female
Newborn	3.0	3.4
3 months	6.3	5.7
6 months	8.1	7.5
9 months	9.2	8.6
1 year	10.2	9.5
18 months	11.4	10.8
2 years	12.0	12
3 years	14.7	14
4 years	16.5	16
5 years	18.6	18
$6^1/_2$ years	22	21.5
$8^1/_2$ years	27	27.2
$10^1/_2$ years	33	34
$12^1/_2$ years	40.2	42.8
$14^1/_2$ years	52	52
$16^1/_2$ years	62.5	56.2

2006). Weigh children, in particular infants, at the same time of the day in relation to their feeding (Hall & Elliman 2003).

Length
(Basic skill)

Length is usually measured in the 0- to 18-month age group. This should be undertaken with an appropriate measuring device and not a tape (Hall & Elliman 2003). Neonates should have their legs extended.

Height
(Basic skill)

From about 2 years of age upwards, height can be measured against an accurate tool.

Head circumference
(Basic skill)

A non-stretch tape (often non-reusable) is used to measure the greatest circumference: around the frontal bones, just above the eyes and over the occipital prominence. Children up to 2 years (and up to 6 years for children developmentally delayed) have this measurement undertaken, as brain growth can be affected by poor nutrition (Klein 1997).

Body mass index (BMI)
(Basic skill)

BMI may be more useful in older children and in young people or for the overweight/obese child. A BMI of <20 may indicate undermalnutrition (Baxter 1999) and over 30, obesity. This measure should be taken into account alongside height and weight. A simple internet search will provide an automated calculation.

$$BMI = \frac{Weight\ (kg)}{Height^2\ (m)}$$

NUTRITIONAL CLINICAL ASSESSMENT
(Basic skill)

- Note if the child has any conditions that may cause nutrient loss, e.g. drains, fistulas, vomiting, diarrhoea, malabsorption syndrome.

- Observe general appearance for over- or underweight, any oedema or pressure areas.
- Assess skin for dry, thin or wrinkled texture, delayed wound healing, poor turgor, oedema.
- Inspect for any signs of infection or sepsis, e.g. wounds, catheter sites, bloodstream.
- Stress and/or non-use of the gut can cause a gut mucosal atrophy, increasing permeability and translocation of bacteria from the gut into the bloodstream, with subsequent septicaemia (Mainous *et al.* 1994).
- Note any diarrhoea or constipation.
- Measure vital signs.
- Undertake respiratory examination (see Chapter 2) and look for:
  - inspiratory and expiratory muscle weakness;
  - decreased lung compliance and atelectasis;
  - rapid, shallow breathing.
- Undertake a cardiovascular examination (see Chapter 4) and look for:
  - bradycardia;
  - hypotension;
  - decreased cardiac output;
  - ECG changes: increased QT interval, decreased voltage.
- Examine the musculoskeletal system (see Chapter 12) for muscle-wasting, short stature, thin legs and arms, abnormal bony prominences (vertebrae, ribcage), wasted buttocks.
- Examine the neurological system (see Chapters 6 and 7) for confusion, irritability, sensory or motor loss.
- Examine the GI system (see Chapter 8) and look for decreased intestine motility and poor feed absorption.
- Observe for altered behaviour including extreme tiredness or lack of interest.
- Note any delayed puberty (sexual development not covered in this book).
- Assess head and neck (see Chapter 11) for:
  - hair that lacks shine, is dry or thinning;
  - eyes that are dull, dry, pale;
  - lips that are red and inflamed or fissured;

    ○ gums that are swollen and bleed easily or are inflamed;
    ○ teeth that are discoloured, have caries;
    ○ tongue that is smooth, swollen, pale, red, painful;
    ○ visible thyroid, palpable outwith the midline position.

OTHER ANTHROPOMETRIC MEASURES
(Advanced skill)
Nutrition specialists may use other tools to gain further information.

Triceps skin fold thickness
This is easily measured with skin fold (constant tension) calipers, to determine muscle mass.

Midarm circumference
This measures body fat content. Use a non-stretchable tape and measure midway between the acromion in the shoulder and olecranon (elbow); it may be useful to repeat three times, ensuring an accurate result (Verger & Schears 2001).

WEIGHT FOR CALCULATING DRUG DOSAGES
Weight is essential for calculating drug dosages in all children. If the child is critically ill, he or she may be nursed on a weighing bed. If this is not available it may not be possible to weigh the child and therefore estimation is required:

- Ask the parents/carers if they have a recent weight.
- Estimate the weight based on the health care practitioner's experience (not best practice).
- Use a tool, e.g.
  ○ Broselow tape: measuring the length of the child gives an approximate associated weight;
  ○ Oakley chart: also relates the length of a child to the weight;
  ○ the following formula: (age (in years) + 4) × 2 (Resuscitation Council (UK) 2004).

Whether ambulatory or in bed, when weighing the sick child:

- subtract the weight of any arm boards, casts, etc.;
- use the same scale at the same time of day;

- non-ambulatory scales may include bed scales or lifting the patient onto scales, e.g. the neonate.

Capillary leak and oedema resulting from critical illness can reduce the effectiveness of weight as an indicator (Verger & Schears 2001).

BIOCHEMICAL INDICES
(Advanced skill)
- Urea level: can indicate decreased protein intake but is an unreliable sign on its own.
- Plasma protein levels: can be a poor indicator in critical illness when proteins are affected by any pathological state; albumin can be a poor indicator as there can be other causes of albumin loss, e.g. losses from drains or stress.
- Transferrin levels: transferrin is synthesised in liver and transports iron in plasma and is sensitive to protein deficiency.
- Urine:
  - creatinine height index (CHI) reflects muscle mass (assuming normal renal function); a 24-hour urine collection can be used to measure creatinine to give an index: a low index suggests a protein malnutrition state (Verger & Schears 2001);
  - urea nitrogen; a 24-hour urine collection estimates nitrogen balance and assesses catabolic state.
- Indirect calorimetry:
  - carbon dioxide (CO_2) and oxygen (O_2) levels in inspired and expired air are measured and compared to determine energy expenditure using an analyser (O_2 and CO_2 production reflect measurements of intracellular metabolism);
  - the inspiratory and expiratory samplers are placed in the ventilator tubing and connected to a computerised terminal (metabolic cart) at the bedside. Results can be affected by different factors (Martinez *et al*. 2004), so check:
    - that the child is at rest
    - that there is no fever
    - how stable the physiological parameters are
    - that there is minimal (<10%) air leak around the ETT

- that the FiO_2 is less than 0.6
- that there are no airway secretions and the child will not require imminent ETT suctioning.

The CO_2/O_2 ratio can determine specific substrate utilisation. A 30-minute measurement can represent a 24-hour period and may only be required to be calculated two to three times per week (Smyrnios *et al.* 1997). The clinical use of this mode is still in its infancy.

DETERMINING ENERGY REQUIREMENTS

The World Health Organisation (1985) and the Department of Health (1991, 2003) have both produced documents and recommendations for normal dietary requirements of infants and children. Table 9.3 outlines the normal energy requirements for infants and children (basic skill). Normal values may be different in your unit. *(Write in your normal values beside those in the table.)*

Stress factors

(Advanced skill)

The hypermetabolism associated with child illness results in higher energy expenditure (EE; normally about 10% above BMR). The extent of the stress reflects the EE and can be increased from 50% in sepsis up to 100% in burns (Pollack 1993). Other activities can also increase EE including:

Table 9.3 Normal daily dietary requirements of infants and children.

Age	kcal/kg/day	kcal/day
0–2 months	115	
2–3 months	100	
4–12 months	95	
1–4 years	95	
5–6 years	85	
7–10 years	65 or	1600–2000 (females less than males)
11–14 years	46 or	1700–2200 (females less than males)

- respiration, e.g. the work of breathing in a child with bronchiolitis may increase EE up to 40 times (Pollack 1993);
- doing a chest X-ray;
- dressing changes.

Therefore increased calories can be administered according to these stress factors. However, this has led to clinically significant, inaccurate predicted energy requirements, often with subsequent overfeeding, and has since been challenged.

- Critically ill children may have a lower than expected EE due to the administration of ventilation, humidification, analgesia or sedation (White *et al*. 2000).
- The use of neuromuscular blockade appears to have either a decrease in EE (Vernon & Witte 2000) or no impact (Briassoulis *et al*. 2000; White *et al*. 2000).
- A raised temperature increases EE (Joosten *et al*. 1999); for every 1°C of fever, an extra 10% of calories may be required.

Predictive equations
(Advanced skill)
These have been developed over the years, but recent literature has challenged their ability to predict EE in critically ill children with acceptable accuracy for clinical use (Martinez *et al*. 2004). Equations include:

- Harris–Benedict: originally adult based (Harris & Benedict 1919)
- Caldwell–Kennedy: paediatric (Caldwell & Kennedy-Caldwell 1981)
- Schofield: paediatric (Schofield 1985)
- FAO/WHO/UN: paediatric (WHO 1985)
- Maffeis: paediatric (Maffeis *et al*. 1993)
- Fleisch: paediatric (Fleisch 1951)
- Kleiber: originally adult based (Kleiber 1975)
- Dreyer: originally adult based (Sherman 1952)
- Hunter: originally adult based (Hunter *et al*. 1988)

(*Note here which equations you might use in your practice:*)

Indirect calorimetry
(Advanced skill)
Because specific substrate utilisation can be determined, the macronutrients, carbohydrate, protein and fat calorie requirements can be calculated more accurately.

NUTRITION DELIVERY
Naso-/orogastric tubes (NGT/OGT)
(Basic skill)
Normally a nasogastric route will be chosen; however, place the tube via the mouth:

- when the child has suffered a head injury (the tube may enter the brain if there is a fractured base of skull);
- in premature infants and neonates (they are obligatory nose breathers).

The stomach is one of the least tolerant areas of the gut and therefore check for:

- feeding intolerance (see below);
- diarrhoea;
- gastro-oesophageal reflux;
- pulmonary aspiration (signs of respiratory distress; see Chapter 2), especially when there is not an intact gag or cough reflex.

Check the position of the tube by:

- X-ray (see Chapter 3) (Metheny & Titler 2001);
- pH: test the aspirate with pH paper or an electronic pH meter (Berry *et al*. 1994; Metheny *et al*. 1998; Colagiovanni 1999; Metheny & Titler 2001). Table 9.4 shows the values of aspirate;
- observing the aspirate: Table 9.5 shows different observations;
- looking in the child's mouth to ensure there is no coiling of the tube;
- noting if the child can vocalise: a tube through the larynx will affect speech.

Table 9.4 Interpretation of gastric tube pH testing.

pH	Interpretation
<4	Tube is likely to be in stomach
<5 and there is use of histamine antagonists or antacids NB: try to test prior to administration of these	Tube is likely to be in stomach
6 or above	Tube is likely to be in the lung or intestine

Table 9.5 Gastric aspirate assessment.

Aspirate	Interpretation
Yellow/clear/with off-white mucus or sediment/feed remains	Typical normal gastric fluid
Green bile	May indicate bowel obstruction
Phlegm-like/white/thick	May indicate respiratory aspirate
Dark colour	May indicate small intestine position

Note that checking aspirate with litmus paper for an acidic reading and using auscultation to check for correct gastric tube placements are no longer recommended and not considered best practice due to their inaccuracy (Methany et al. 1994, 1998; Neuman et al. 1995).

If no aspirate can be retrieved, try:

- checking the length of the tube that has been inserted;
- pushing 3–10 ml of air into the tube to push the tube away from the stomach wall;
- changing the position of the child so that the lumen of the tube moves;
- offering the child a drink (if appropriate) to increase stomach fluid volume;
- waiting for 30 minutes and then rechecking;
- reviewing local guidelines – to discuss with colleagues, or consider an X-ray.

Nasojejunal tubes (NJT) or post-pyloric feeding
(Advanced skill)

These tubes are used for feeding when the small intestine may be functional even if the stomach is not (Raper & Maynard 1992). Nutrition can be continued via an NJT throughout the weaning and extubation of the endotracheal tube process (Lyons *et al.* 2002). They may also be used for the child with a gastro-oesophageal reflux (Meyer *et al.* 2001).

The NJT can be difficult to position and the child may need a general anaesthetic or sedation and a fluoroscopy/endosopy procedure with a follow-up X-ray confirmation of position. However, bedside placement has been described with a high degree of success (Meyer *et al.* 2001) and is outlined in Table 9.6.

Securing the nasogastric/nasojejunal tube
(Basic skill)
- Ensure the skin is clean.
- Apply a skin protectant (e.g. an adhesive pad or a special skin preparation) to the cheek/nose.
- Apply tape
  - to the nose (in older children)
  - to the cheek (in younger children and infants).
- Use a commercially available attachment device.
- Check the skin integrity of the nare (see Chapter 14).

Gastrostomy
(Advanced skill)

A gastrostomy may be a balloon or skin level gastrostomy. It is a surgical opening into the stomach through the abdominal wall for long-term feeding; it may also be performed percutaneously (percutaneous endoscopic gastrostomy – PEG). A tube may be inserted within the PEG to feed into the jejunum (PEG-J). Jejunostomies may also be performed where direct feeding to the jejunum is performed.

General care of the gastrostomy site
Issues for assessment, using local protocols include (Holden *et al.* 1997):

Table 9.6 Placement of a naso-jejunal tube.

Procedure

- Use a non-weighted tube and lubricate the guidewire
- Mark out the length of tube required: from the nose to the ear, down to the umbilicus and finally to the right iliac crest
- Position the child on the left lateral and raise the bed to 15–30°
- Empty the stomach via the naso-gastric tube already in place
- Take the tip of the tube and lubricate it before gently pushing it horizontally through the nare (same side as naso-gastric tube) and naso-pharynx until it reaches the stomach
- Check any aspirate from the stomach with pH paper (if it is 4–5 then confirmation of placement is achieved); if aspiration is undertaken flush the tube with water before advancing further, ensuring no stomach contents remain in the tube
- Keep pushing the tube in slowly, using a rotation movement at the nostril
- There may be some resistance at the pylorus
- Once the measured length of the tube has been inserted, use a stethoscope to listen at a point between the umbilicus and iliac crest whilst air is injected into the tube; you should be able to hear the sound of air being injected clearly

Hints and tips

- If the tube jumps back towards you when you let it go, it may mean that it is bent or twisted and blocked inside; in which case, pull it back and start again
- A prokinetic agent (erythromycin, metoclopramide) may assist when first and second attempts fail (watch for side effects of these drugs)
- Remove the guidewire carefully as the tube may accidentally be withdrawn with it; remove once the need for a scan (to check placement) is no longer required

Methylene blue test to confirm placement without the need for an X-ray

- Mix 0.1 ml methylene blue with 20 ml water or feed and insert the following amount into the tube:
  ○ 20 ml for the child over 15 kg
  ○ 10 ml for the child between 5 and 15 kg
  ○ 5 ml for the child less than 5 kg
- Aspirate the *naso*-gastric tube 10 minutes later and check for absence of methylene blue solution; discard all the solution

- Site cleaning: usually daily site cleansing using non-touch technique until well healed (4–6 weeks), then site may be cleansed as part of normal daily bathing/showering routine. A cotton bud may be useful. Fixation devices may occasionally need to be removed for cleansing; seek specialist advice to undertake this risky procedure.

- Observe for signs of infection: check for any inflammation (redness, swelling, pain), abnormal discharge or odour.
- Accidental decannulation: ensure an appropriate-size catheter is available to insert into the stoma. Do not use this tube as a feeding tube until its position has been checked and assured.
- Balloon care: change sterile water in the balloon (usually 5 ml) weekly to ensure patency of balloon.
- Manipulation of the fixation device: rotate the device 360° daily to prevent adherence to the skin.
- Feeding regimes/drug administration: see 'Nutrition Delivery' above. Check that any medication prescribed is a suitable preparation for gastrostomy administration.

METHODS OF FEED ADMINISTRATION
Bolus feeding
(Basic skill)
Bolus feeding:

- provides a more normal gastric loading;
- is not used for jejunal feeding as a reservoir is not available;
- can give rise to stomach cramps, regurgitation, diarrhoea or an increase in BMR;
- is often used as a staging from continuous feeding to normal oral feeding regime;
- is used as a short-term measure in acutely ill children;
- can be used in chronic long-term illness, e.g. cystic fibrosis.

Continuous feeding
(Basic skill)
- Continuous feeding is used with jejunal feeding to ensure low-flow delivery.
- It can reduce abdominal distension, nausea and vomiting, and diarrhoea.
- The thermogenic effect of feeding may be lost, so nutrition is more energy efficient.
- Insulin effect may be reduced (Beau & Labat 1994).

- Due to the pH not returning to normal, the stomach may be colonised; if gag and cough reflexes are not intact, slow aspiration of feeds can cause a nosocomial pneumonia (Horwood 1992; Skiest 1996).
- An 8-hour break is recommended; however, due to the potential for hypoglycaemia, 4-hour breaks are more usual – these need to be organised to best meet the needs of the child, e.g. overnight for hospitalised children, during the day for children at home, to facilitate weaning and extubation of intensive care children.
- There may be a higher incidence of blocked tubes (Ciocon 1992).
- Check any tube-administered medication prescriptions for administration requirements; they may need rest periods before or after administration.

Changing feeding sets
(Basic skill)
- Using a clean, non-touch technique, assemble all equipment and fill with 24-hours' worth of feed (Patchell *et al.* 1998).
- Change every 24 hours unless otherwise directed by manufacturer.
- Local policies will guide practice for length of time feed can be disconnected before reconnecting to patients (usually 4 hours).

(Write your clinical unit guidelines here:)

Which feed
(Advanced skill)
Where possible, breast milk is the choice of milk feed for infants. Feeds are given at full strength. Some examples of formula feeds include:

- Infants: SMA (67 kcal/100 ml)
- Toddlers – school age: Paediasure or Nutrini (1 kcal/ml)
- Over 6 years: Osmolite or Jevity (1 kcal/ml)

(Note here which ready-made feeds are available in your practice area for different age groups:)

FEED ADDITIVES
(Advanced skill)
- Thickening agents: may be required for those infants who have a gastro-oesophageal reflux.
- Glucose polymer may be added for those infants who are failing to thrive.

MONITORING DURING FEEDING
Check the tube
(Basic skill)
- Check for date of insertion, size and type; consider if it needs changing due to local policy, e.g. PVC tubes every 14 days and polyurethane (fine bore) tubes every 28 days. For longer-term use a Ryles tube may need to be replaced with a fine bore tube.

(*Write your clinical unit policy here:*)

- Check for position and migration – there is a high rate of tube malposition in children (Ellett *et al*. 1998):
  - mark or note the correct position of the tube;
  - check pH of aspirate before each feed or medication administration and 12 hourly when on continuous feeds (see 'Naso-/orogastric tubes (NGT/OGT)' above).
- Check for blockage: prevent by aspirating and flushing the tube with 2–5 ml of water:
  - prior to and after each feed;
  - prior to and after each medication administration;
  - regularly in continuous feeding (e.g. every 4–6 hours);
  - if actually blocked use:
    - warm water (5–10 ml depending on age of child) and a push–pull motion to try to unblock the tube; the larger the syringe used in aspiration, the less pressure is exerted on the tube and therefore a 50-ml syringe is recommended;
    - a little fizzy water or sodium bicarbonate mixed with water (a 5% solution);
    - commercially available products.

Check the feed
(Basic skill)
- Check that it has been out of the refrigerator for at least 30 minutes prior to administration.
- Calculate the prescribed volume of feed (each shift) and ensure that what is prescribed is actually administered within the 24 hours; see fluid calculations in Chapter 10.
- Check the feed has been commenced as soon as possible, unless contraindicated, and ideally within 6 hours of admission (Adams 1994) to reduce stress response and encourage gut motility.
- Calculate nutrient intake (each shift) and determine if total daily nutritional requirements are being met.

  For example: a 1-month-old 4-kg baby requires 115 kcal/kg/day
  > SMA is being used (0.67 kcal/ml)
  > Kilocalories required = $4 \times 115 = 460$
  > SMA volume required = $460 \times 0.67 = 308$ ml/day

Note that 'full feeds' means that the *total* daily nutritional requirements are being met, not that the prescription has been met.

Check the pump
(Basic skill)
- Ideally a specific feed administration pump should be used, e.g. Kangaroo/Patrol pump.
- If using an IV infusion device pump, effective and clear labelling must be unambiguous; always consider how someone else can easily identify the feeding tube and pump.
- Check what has been dialled up is actually being administered, especially when using thickened feeds; you may want to use a burette in the feeding set to measure actual intake (Philip Wilson, personal communication, 2005).

Check the patient
(Basic skill)
- Nurse head-up to reduce the incidence of aspiration.
- Undertake anthropometric measures regularly, as determined to be appropriate in your practice, e.g. weigh weekly.

- Monitor blood liver function, urea and electrolyte, glucose, haemoglobin and urine electrolytes daily or as appropriate.
- Monitor bedside blood glucose 4–24 hourly, as appropriate.
- Check regular normal bowel habits.
- Assess the need for prokinetics.
- Document fluid input and output.

Commencing feeds at an appropriate time, preventing interruption of feeding, e.g. through blockage of tubes or ill-timed procedures, and managing tolerance can be determined through the use of a guideline or flowchart. Figure 9.1 shows one such example.

TOLERATING FEEDS
(Basic skill)
Assess the following factors when judging tolerance of feeding:

- Diarrhoea:
  - Assess the potential causes; could be caused by many things including antibiotics, infection, high osmolar feeds, medications.
  - Could be part of 'dumping syndrome' when feeds are too cold or too quickly administered (often associated with jejunal feeding); symptoms include:
    - diarrhoea
    - cramping/abdominal pain
    - weakness
    - light-headedness
    - palpitations
    - diaphoresis (sweating).
- Abdominal distension: ensure the distension is not just due to air alone; aspirate the stomach.
- Abdominal pain and tenderness.
- Nausea and vomiting: assess other potential causes, e.g. head injury or medications.
- Large aspirates:
  - What constitutes a large aspirate or residual volume needs to be determined at a local level, e.g.

- the volume greater than the amount of feed given since the last assessment (Taylor 1989);
- aspirates from 5 ml/kg up to 150 ml in total (Taylor & Baker 1999a,b).

o The volume of aspirate does not necessarily mean intolerance of feed and consequently feeding should not be stopped unless coupled with other signs of intolerance, as discussed above (McClave 1992).

o Assess the content of the aspirate for state of digestion: curdled-type aspirate suggests some gastro-intestinal tract function and bile aspirates may suggest bowel obstruction.

o Return aspirates to the child, as fluid and electrolyte imbalances may occur with discarding it (Hazinski 1992).

Local policy will influence practice, especially with paucity of recent evidence.

(Note your clinical unit policy here:)

OVERFEEDING
(Basic skill)
Due to the inaccuracy of predicting energy requirements, monitor for overfeeding by checking for:

- diarrhoea;
- hydration state (see Chapter 10);
- hyperglycaemia: can cause osmotic diuresis and enhance bacterial growth (Elia 1995);
- glycosuria;
- weight gain;
- fatty liver and liver dysfunction: check blood liver function tests;
- electrolyte imbalances: check blood electrolyte levels;
- signs of increased oxygen demand:
  o respiratory distress and failure (see Chapter 2)
  o acidosis (see Chapter 3)
  o tachycardia (see Chapter 4).

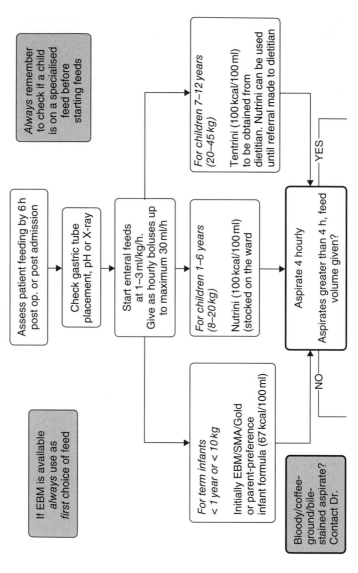

Fig. 9.1 Great Ormond Street Hospital for Children NHS Trust protocol for feeding using nasogastric/gastrostomy tubes for children with normal renal function in the paediatric intensive care unit (PICU). (Reproduced with slight amendment.)

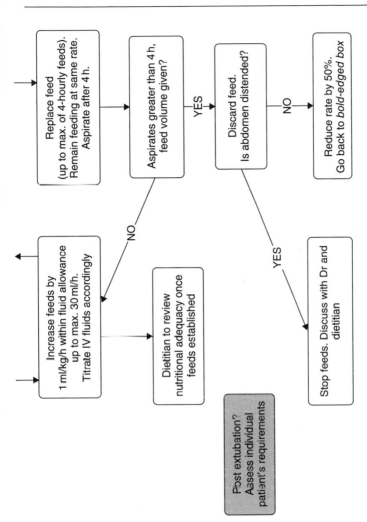

Fig. 9.1 *Continued.*

225

SUMMARY

Health care professionals have a responsibility to undertake an appropriate nutritional assessment, formulate a feeding plan and evaluate it. Depending on the clinical setting, a range of assessment techniques can be used. Interruption to feeding regimes should be minimised and tolerance of feed must be continually evaluated.

REFERENCES

Adam, S.K. (1994) Aspects of current research in enteral nutrition in the critically ill. *Care of the Critically Ill*, **10** (6), 246–251.

Baxter, J.P. (1999) Problems of nutritional assessment in the acute setting. *Proceedings of the Nutrition Society*, **58**, 39–46.

Beau, P. & Labat, J. (1994) Continuous vs. discontinuous enteral nutrition: compared effects on serum lipoproteins in humans. *Journal of Parenteral and Enteral Nutrition*, **18** (4), 331–334.

Berry, S., Schoettker, P. & Orr, M. (1994) pH measurements as a guide for establishing short-term postpyloric enteral access. *Nutrition*, **10** (5), 419–423.

Briassoulis, G., Venkataraman, S. & Thompson, A. (2000) Energy expenditure in critically ill children. *Critical Care Medicine*, **28** (4), 1166–1172.

British Association for Parenteral and Enteral Nutrition (BAPEN) (2005) *Malnutrition Screening Tool* (MUST). BAPEN, Redditch.

Caldwell, M.D. & Kennedy-Caldwell, C. (1981) Normal nutritional requirements. *Surgical Clinics of North America*, **61**, 489–506.

Child Growth Foundation (1996a) *Girls Four-in-One Growth Charts*. Child Growth Foundation, London.

Child Growth Foundation (1996b) *Boys Four-in-One Growth Charts*. Child Growth Foundation, London.

Chinn, S. (1996) Growth charts for ethnic populations in the UK. *The Lancet*, **347**, 839–840.

Ciocon, J.O. (1992) Continuous compared with intermittent tube feeding in the elderly. *Journal of Parenteral and Enteral Nutrition*, **16** (6), 525–528.

Colagiovanni, L. (1999) Taking the tube. *Nursing Times*, **95** (21), 63–70.

Cole, T.J. (1994) Do growth chart centiles need a face lift? *British Medical Journal*, **308**, 641–642.

Cross, J.H., Holden, C., Pearmain, G., Stevens, M.C.G. & Booth, I.W. (1995) Clinical examination compared with anthropometry in evaluating nutritional status. *Archives of Disease in Childhood*, **72**, 60–61.

Department of Health (1991) *Dietary Reference Values for Food Energy and Nutrients for the United Kingdom* (Report 41). HMSO, London.

Department of Health (2003) NHS *Immunisation Statistics*. Available at http://www.dh.gov.uk/Policy/ions/topics.

Department of Health (2004a) *The National Service Frameworks for Children, Young People and Maternity Services*. DH, London.

Department of Health (2004b) *Standards For Better Health*. DH, London.

Ekvall, S.W., Ekvall, V.K., Walberg-Wolfe, J. & Nehring, W. (2005) Nutritional assessment – all levels and ages. In: Ekvall, S.W. & Ekvall, V.K. (eds) *Pediatric Nutrition in Chronic Diseases and Developmental Disorders: Prevention, Assessment and Treatment*, 2nd edn. Oxford University Press, Oxford.

Elia, M. (1995) Changing concepts of nutrition requirements in disease: implications for artificial nutritional support. *The Lancet*, **345**, 1279–1284.

Ellett, M.L.C., Maahs, J. & Forsee, S. (1998) Prevalence of feeding tube placement errors and associated risk factors in children. *Maternal Child Health Nursing*, **23** (5), 234–239.

Fleisch, A. (1951) Le metabolisme basal standard et sa détermination au moyen du 'Metabocalculator'. *Helvetia Medica Acta*, **18**, 23–45.

Freeman, J.V., Cole, T.J., Chinn, S., Jones, P.R.M., White, E.M. & Preece, M.A. (1995) Cross-sectional stature and weight reference curves for the UK, 1990. *Archives of Diseases in Childhood*, **73**, 17–24.

Gaw, A., Cowan, R.A., O'Reilly, D., Stewart, M.J. & Shepherd, J. (1999) *Clinical Biochemistry*, 2nd edn. Churchill Livingston, Edinburgh.

Great Ormond Street Hospital for Children NHS Trust (2000) *Nutritional Requirements for Children in Health and Disease*. Great Ormond Street Hospital, London.

Hall, D. & Elliman, D. (2003) *Health For All Children*, 4th edn. Oxford University Press, New York.

Harris, J.A. & Benedict, F.G. (1919) *Standard Basal Metabolism Constants for Physiologists and Clinicians: A Biometric Study of Basal Metabolism in Man*. Carnegie Institute, Philadelphia.

Hazinski, M.F. (1992) *Nursing Care of the Critically Ill Child*, 2nd edn. Mosby Year Book, St. Louis.

Hendrikse, W.H., Reilly, J.J. & Weaver, L.T. (1997) Malnutrition in a children's hospital. *Clinical Nutrition*, **16**, 13–18.

Holden, C., Sexton, E. & Paul, L. (1997) Enteral nutrition for children. *Nursing Standard*, **11** (32), 49–54.

Horwood, A. (1992) A literature review of recent advances in enteral feeding and the increased understanding of the gut. *Intensive and Critical Care Nursing*, **8**, 185–188.

Hunter, D.C., Jaksic, T. & Lewis, D. (1988) Resting energy expenditure in the critically ill: estimation versus measurement. *British Journal of Surgery*, **75**, 875–878.

Joosten, K.F., Verhoeven, J., Hop, W. & Hazelzet, J. (1999) Indirect calorimetry in mechanically ventilated infants and children: accuracy of total daily energy expenditure with 2 hour measurements. *Clinical Nutrition*, **18** (3), 149–152.

Kleiber, M. (1975) *The Fire of the Life*. Huntingdon, New York.

Klein, S. (1997) Nutrition support in clinical practice: review of published data and recommendations for future research directions. *American Journal of Clinical Nutrition*, **66**, 683–706.

Lyons, K.L., Brilli, R.J., Wieman, R.A. & Jacobs, B.R. (2002) Continuation of transpyloric feeding during weaning of mechanical ventilation and tracheal extubation in children: a randomised controlled trial. *Journal of Parenteral and Enteral Nutrition*, **26** (3), 209–216.

Maffeis, C., Schutz, Y. & Micciolo, R. (1993) Resting metabolic rate in six- to ten-year-old obese and non-obese children. *Journal of Pediatrics*, **122**, 556–562.

Mainous, M.R., Block, E.F.J. & Deitch, E.A. (1994) Nutritional support of the gut: how and why. *New Horizons*, **2** (2), 193–201.

Martinez, J.L.V., Martinez-Romillo, P.D., Sebastion, J.D. & Tarrio, F.R. (2004) Predicted versus measured energy expenditure by continuous, online indirect calorimetry in ventilated, critically ill children during the early postinjury period. *Pediatric Critical Care Medicine*, **5** (1), 19–27.

McClave, S.A. (1992) Use of residual volume as a marker for enteral feeding tolerance: prospective blinded comparison with physical examination and radiographic findings. *Journal of Parenteral and Enteral Nutrition*, **16** (2), 99–105.

Metheny, N.A. & Titler, M.G. (2001) Assessing placement of feeding tubes. *American Journal of Nursing*, **101** (5), 36–46.

Metheny, N.A., Clouse, R.E., Clark, J.M., Reed, L., Wehrle, M.A. & Wiersema, L. (1994) pH testing of feeding tube aspirates to determine placement. *Nutrition in Clinical Practice*, **9** (5), 185–190.

Metheny, N.A., McSweeney, M., Wehrle, M.A. & Wiersema, A. (1998) Effectiveness of the auscultatory method in predicting feeding tube location. *Nursing Research*, **39** (5), 262–267.

Meyer, R., Harrison, S. & Mehta, C. (2001) Bedside placement of nasojejunal tubes in children. *Care of the Critically Ill*, How To Guide.

National Institute for Health and Clinical Excellence (NICE) (2006) *Nutrition Support in Adults, Clinical Guideline 32.* NICE, London.

Neumann, R.J., Meyer, C.T., Dutton, J.L. & Smith, R. (1995) Hold that X-ray: aspirate pH and auscultation prove enteral tube placement. *Journal of Clinical Gastroenterology,* **20** (4), 293–295.

NHS Modernisation Agency (2003) *Essence of Care Patient-Focused Benchmarks for Clinical Governance.* DH, London.

Patchell, C.J., Anderson, A. & Holden, C. (1998) Reducing bacterial contamination of enteral feeds. *Archives of Disease in Childhood,* **78**, 166–168.

Pollack, M. (1993) Nutritional support of children in the intensive care unit. In: Suskind, R. & Lewinter-Suskind, L. (eds) *Textbook of Pediatric Nutrition,* 2nd edn. Raven Press, New York.

Raper, S. & Maynard, N. (1992) Feeding the critically ill patient. *British Journal of Nursing,* **1** (6), 273–280.

Resuscitation Council (UK) (2004) *European Paediatric Life Support Course Provider Manual.* Resuscitation Council (UK), London.

Royal College of Nursing (2006) Malnutrition in children and young people: what nurses working with children need to know and do. An RCN position statement. Available at www.rcn.org.uk.

Schofield, W.N. (1985) Predicting basal metabolic rate: new standards and review of previous work. *Human Nutrition, Clinical Nutrition,* **39** (Suppl. C), 5–41.

Sherman, H.C. (1952) *Chemistry of Food and Nutrition,* 8th edn. Macmillan, New York.

Skiest, D. (1996) The role of enteral feeding in gastric colonisation: a randomised controlled trial comparing continuous to intermittent enteral feeding in mechanically ventilated patients. *Clinical Intensive Care,* **7**, 138–143.

Smyrnios, N.A., Curley, F.J. & Shaker, K.G. (1997) Accuracy of 30-minute indirect calorimetry studies in predicting 24-hour energy expenditure in mechanically ventilated, critically ill patients. *Journal of Parenteral and Enteral Nutrition,* **21**, 168–174.

Taylor, R. & Baker, A. (1999a) Enteral nutrition in critical illness: part one. *Paediatric Nursing,* **11** (7), 16–20.

Taylor, R. & Baker, A. (1999b) Enteral nutrition in critical illness: part two. *Paediatric Nursing,* **11** (8), 26–31.

Taylor, S. (1989) Preventing complications in enteral feeding. *Professional Nurse,* February, 247–249.

Thomas, B. (1994) *The Manual of Dietetic Practice,* 2nd edn. Blackwell, Oxford.

Verger, J. & Schears, G. (2001) Nutrition support. In: Curley, M.A.Q. & Moloney-Harmon, P.A. (eds) *Critical Care Nursing of Infants and Children,* 2nd edn. W.B. Saunders, Philadelphia.

Vernon, D. & Witte, M. (2000) Effect of neuromuscular blockade on oxygen consumption and energy expenditure in sedated, mechanically ventilated children. *Critical Care Medicine*, **28** (5), 1569–1571.

White, M., Shepherd, R. & McEniery, J. (2000) Energy expenditure in 100 ventilated, critically ill children: improving the accuracy of predictive equations. *Critical Care Medicine*, **28** (7), 2307–2312.

World Health Organisation (1985) *Energy and Protein Requirements: Report of a Joint FAO/WHO/UNU Expert Consultation.* WHO Technical Report Series no. 724, Geneva.

Fluid and Electrolytes

INTRODUCTION

There is a variable total body water (TBW) percentage per body weight among different child age groups as well as changes in distribution of the intracellular and extracellular compartments, e.g. the extracellular fluid (ECF) reduces from 50% of body weight at birth to 30% by 2 years of age. Water and electrolyte disturbances occur rapidly in children, particularly young children and infants (Lam 1998). Larger amounts of fluid can be lost through the large body surface area. There is a higher metabolic rate and therefore more waste to excrete, and in infancy, the kidney is immature, concentrating urine less effectively (Wong 1995). Small changes in fluid loss can have a large impact (Lorenz 1997). The aim of this chapter is to outline the assessment techniques of fluid and electrolytes.

LEARNING OBJECTIVES

By the end of this chapter the reader will be able to:

❑ Understand normal electrolyte values and requirements.
❑ Assess the hydration status of the child.
❑ Calculate appropriate fluid requirements.
❑ Assess indwelling catheters.
❑ Evaluate fluid balance.
❑ Understand the need for blood glucose assessment and administration.

NORMAL ELECTROLYTE AND GLUCOSE LEVELS AND DAILY REQUIREMENTS

Table 10.1 shows normal serum electrolyte levels and normal daily requirements in one unit. (*Write in the normal levels for your clinical area, as these may be slightly different.*)

Table 10.1 Normal serum electrolyte levels and daily requirements.

Electrolyte	Normal serum levels (mmol/L)	Normal for your practice	Normal daily requirements	Normal for your practice
Potassium (K⁺)	3.5–5		2 mmol/kg/day	
Sodium (Na²⁺)	136–146		3 mmol/kg/day	
Calcium (Ca²⁺)	Infant 1.74–3 Child 2.2–2.7		1 mmol/kg/day	
Chloride (Chl⁻)	95–105		2 mmol/kg/day	
Glucose	Neonate 1.7–3.3 Child 3.3–5.5		10% for neonates 5–10% for infants	

Table 10.2 outlines clinical signs and ECG abnormalities of common electrolyte imbalances (Park 2002) (advanced skill).

FLUID STATUS
Assess the hydration status of the child (Lam 1998) (basic skill).

Skin turgor
- Gently pinch a roll of skin and roll between fingers.
- Release and watch for its immediate return to normal position.

Normal	Mild dehydration	Moderate dehydration	Severe dehydration
Immediate return	Immediate return	Slow return	Very slow return

- Delay in return will cause 'tenting' of the skin.

Oedema
- Look for shiny, tight skin.
- Press gently over affected area for 5 seconds and release; look for pitting.

Table 10.2 Clinical signs and ECG findings of common electrolyte disturbances.

Electrolyte imbalance	Clinical signs	ECG findings
Hypokalaemia	Muscle weakness Lethargy/irritable Nausea/vomiting	T waves are inverted/ flattened
Hyperkalaemia	Muscle weakness Confusion Nausea/vomiting	Tall peaked T waves with progressively widening QRS complexes, then ventricular arrhythmias
Hyponatraemia	Lethargy and disorientation – may progress to fitting and coma Muscle cramps Nausea/vomiting	
Hypernatraemia	Irritable/lethargic Increased muscle tone – may progress to coma	
Hypocalcaemia	Tingling sensation in hands/ fingers or around the mouth Muscle cramps Lethargy – may progress to seizures May get a hypotension	QT interval is prolonged
Hypercalcaemia	Lethargy – may progress to seizures and coma Nausea/vomiting	QT interval is shortened

- In the infant, oedema is often found in the sacral, peri-orbital or flank areas.
- In the older child, oedema is often found in the extremities.
- Extreme oedema may also be found in the testicle or labia regions.
- Oedema can indicate fluid overload.

Fontanelle (infants)
- Gently palpate the anterior fontanelle with finger tips.
- A soft and flat fontanelle is normal.

Normal	Mild dehydration	Moderate dehydration	Severe dehydration
Soft and flat	Soft and flat	Depressed or sunken	Very depressed

- Any bulging can indicate:
  - overhydration
  - increased intracranial pressure
  - baby crying or vomiting.

Mucous membranes
- Observe the mouth and tongue for moistness.

Normal	Mild dehydration	Moderate dehydration	Severe dehydration
Moist	Moist	Dry	Extremely dry

Eyes
- Observe eyes for brightness and normal position in the eye socket.
- Observe whether tears evident.

Normal	Mild dehydration	Moderate dehydration	Severe dehydration
Bright eyes and normal position Tears	Bright eyes and normal position Tears	Dull eyes slightly sunken Tears absent	Extreme sunkenness Tears absent

Neurological state (see Chapter 7)
- Observe child/infant for normal energetic state.

Normal	Mild dehydration	Moderate dehydration	Severe dehydration
Normal energy levels	Decreased energy	Weak cry and lethargy	Drowsy, decreased level of consciousness

Cardiac/vital signs (see Chapter 4)
- Palpate the pulses for normal rate and volume.
- Perform blood pressure and check for normal values.

Normal	Mild dehydration	Moderate dehydration	Severe dehydration
Normal heart rate and volume	Normal heart rate and volume	Tachycardia and/or weak pulses	Higher tachycardia and very weak pulses
Normal blood pressure	Normal blood pressure	Normal blood pressure	Low blood pressure

- A low blood pressure in children is an ominous sign and management must start immediately (Resuscitation Council (UK) 2004).
- A gallop rhythm may indicate volume overload.

Respiratory (see Chapter 2)
- Check the respiratory rate is normal for the child.
- Auscultate breath sounds.

Normal	Mild dehydration	Moderate dehydration	Severe dehydration
Normal respiratory rate	Normal respiratory rate	Slight hyperpnoea	Fast and deep respiratory pattern

- Crackles or crepitations on auscultation may indicate fluid overload.

Vascular (see Chapter 4)
- Check capillary refill time (CRT) is less than 2 seconds.

Normal	Mild dehydration	Moderate dehydration	Severe dehydration
CRT < 2 seconds	CRT < 2 seconds	CRT > 2 seconds	CRT > 3 seconds

(Roberts 2001)

Renal
- Note the number of dry nappies/amount of urine output.

> Normal urine output:
>   Children: >1 ml/kg/h
>   Infants: 1–2 ml/kg/h
>   Neonates: 2 ml/kg/h (less ability to concentrate urine)

Normal	Mild dehydration	Moderate dehydration	Severe dehydration
Normal urine output volume	Slightly decreased urine output volume	Oliguria (decreased urine output)	Anuria (absent urine output)

Liver
- Hepatomegaly (see Chapter 8) may indicate fluid overload.

Weight
- Weigh the child and note any weight loss or gain.

Normal	Mild dehydration	Moderate dehydration	Severe dehydration
Normal weight gain	5% weight loss	5–10% weight loss	10% weight loss

- Note an increase in weight that may indicate overhydration.

Classification of dehydration I
(Basic skill)

> *Mild*: 5% weight loss plus 'mild' signs above.
> *Moderate*: 5–10% weight loss plus 'moderate' signs above.
> *Severe*: 10% weight loss plus 'severe' signs above.

(Gill & O'Brien 2002)

- Calculating fluid deficit (advanced skill):
  - % dehydrated × weight (kg) × 10 (American Association of Critical Care Nurses 2001);
  - an increase or decrease of temperature: for every 1°C temperature rise or fall, fluid requirements are increased or decreased by 7% (Stack & Dobbs 2004).
- Hypovolaemia can occur due to:
  - fluid loss: vomiting and diarrhoea or increased insensible loss (hyperventilation, sweating, hyperthermia);
  - fluid shift: loss of fluid into third-spaces (pleura, peritoneum, GI tract) in critical illness;
  - decreased intake: nil by mouth.

Classification of dehydration II (O'Callaghan & Stephenson 2002)
(Advanced skill)
Hyponatraemic: low serum sodium levels (<136 mmol/L) mean that more sodium than fluids has been lost. Assess for:

- signs of severe dehydration;
- coma;
- or that too much water has been administered.

Isotonic: serum sodium level is normal, meaning that equal amounts of sodium and fluid are lost. Assess for:

- signs of moderate to severe dehydration.

Hypertonic: serum sodium level is high (>146 mmol/L), meaning that more fluid has been lost than sodium. As a consequence, water will be shifted from the cells to the intravascular compartment. Assess for:

- signs of moderate dehydration;
- severe cerebral irritability (may include fitting);
- muscular hypertonicity (see Chapter 6);
- fair skin turgor.

FLUID ADMINISTRATION
Calculation of normal daily maintenance fluid
(Basic skill)

$$100\,ml/kg \text{ for the first } 10\,kg$$
$$+$$
$$50\,ml/kg \text{ for the second } 10\,kg$$
$$+$$
$$25\,ml/kg \text{ for the remaining kilogramme}$$
$$=$$
$$\text{total daily fluid maintenance requirement}$$

To calculate an hourly rate, divide the daily requirement by 24.

For example: the daily maintenance requirements for a 22-kg child are 1550 ml:

$$100 \times 10 = 1000$$
$$+$$
$$50 \times 10 = 500$$
$$+$$
$$25 \times 2 = 50$$
$$=$$
$$1550\,ml$$

The hourly rate will be 64.58 ml/h or 65 ml/h:

$$\frac{1550}{24} = 64.58$$

Other equations can be used (*write in here any equations you use in your clinical practice:*).

Calculation of partial daily maintenance fluid
(Basic skill)

$$\frac{\text{100\% of total daily fluid (as calculated above)}}{100} \times \text{the percentage of daily requirements}$$

To calculate an hourly rate, divide the daily requirement by 24.

For example: a 22-kg child requiring 80% of daily fluid maintenance needs 1240 ml:

$$\frac{1550}{100} \times 80 = 1240 \text{ ml}$$

The hourly rate will be 51.66 ml/h or 52 ml/h:

$$\frac{1240}{24} = 51.66$$

Calculation of normal hourly maintenance fluid
(Basic skill)

4 ml/kg for the first 10 kg
+
2 ml/kg for the second 10 kg
+
1 ml/kg for the remaining kilogramme
=
fluid requirement in millilitres per hour

For example: a 22-kg child requires:

$4 \times 10 = 40$
+
$2 \times 10 = 20$
+
$1 \times 2 = 2$
=
62 ml/h

Other equations may be used (*write in here any that you use in your practice:*).

Calculation of hourly prescription rate (ml/kg)
(Basic skill)

$$\frac{\text{Prescription rate} \times \text{weight}}{24} = \text{hourly rate}$$

For example: a 25-kg child who has been prescribed 70 ml/kg will need 73 ml/h:

$$\frac{70 \times 25}{24} = 72.91 \text{ ml/h or } 73 \text{ ml/h}$$

Calculation of hourly rate when millilitres per metre squared have been prescribed
(Advanced skill)

$$\frac{\text{ml} \times \text{m}^2}{24} = \text{hourly rate}$$

First the metres squared needs calculating. You will need:

- a nomogram (a chart where you can plot height and weight and get the value) or
- a calculator (with a square root ($\sqrt{}$) symbol)

$$\text{m}^2 = \frac{\sqrt{} \text{ of height} \times \text{weight}}{3600}$$

Calculate by:

- height × weight
- divide by 3600
- press the square root ($\sqrt{}$) symbol

For example: a 15-kg child who is 75 cm long is prescribed 900 ml/m²/day

$$\frac{\text{m}^2}{3600} = \sqrt{} \text{ of } 15 \times 75$$
$$15 \times 75 = 1125$$
$$1125 \div 3600 = 0.3125$$
$$\sqrt{} \text{ of } 0.3125 = 0.5590$$

Then for the hourly rate:

$$\frac{900 \times 0.5590}{24} = 20.96 \,\text{ml/h} \text{ or } 21\,\text{ml/h}$$

Calculating electrolyte maintenance fluid solutions

(Advanced skill)

Intravenous (IV) fluids may take the form of ready-made electrolyte solutions, e.g. a dextrose/saline bag or Hartmann's solution. If a maintenance infusion is required whereby electrolytes are added to a dextrose only solution, the following calculation can be used:

$$\frac{\text{Weight} \times \text{millimoles of electrolyte} \times \text{volume of fluid}}{\text{daily fluid requirements}}$$

where:

- weight of the child is in kilogrammes;
- millimoles of electrolyte is the amount of electrolyte needed per kilogramme per day (this may or may not be 'normal' requirements);
- volume of fluid is the amount of fluid the electrolytes will be added to, e.g. it may be 100 ml (burette) or 500 ml (bag);
- daily fluid requirements need to be calculated (using calculations above) and then any feed volumes or other infusion volumes need to be subtracted.

NB. When calculating these infusions (and indeed any drug calculations) check the final concentrations against the hospital drug formulary (e.g. British National Formulary (BNF 2007)) as these may exceed safety levels for peripheral administration and require a central line for administration.

For example: a 12-kg child will require 80% of daily fluid requirements and is receiving half of this as nasogastric feed. There is also a morphine infusion being administered at 1 ml/h. It has been determined that normal daily requirements of electrolytes (see Table 10.1) are required. The electrolytes are to be put into a burette totalling 100 ml to be *administered via a central line* (too concentrated for a peripheral line).

- Using the calculations above, the daily fluid requirement is 880 ml.
- Half of this will be used in the feeds, leaving 440 ml.
- The morphine infusion of 24 ml in the day leaves 416 ml.
- Once the burette has had electrolytes added to it and has been made up to 100 ml, the hourly IV rate will be 17.3 ml.

Potassium to be added to the burette

$$\frac{12 \times 2 \times 100}{416} = 5.769 \text{ mmol or } 5.8 \text{ mmol}$$

Sodium to be added to the burette

$$\frac{12 \times 3 \times 100}{416} = 8.653 \text{ mmol or } 8.6 \text{ mmol}$$

Calcium to be added to the burette

$$\frac{12 \times 1 \times 100}{416} = 2.884 \text{ mmol or } 2.9 \text{ mmol}$$

Chloride to be added to the burette

$$\frac{12 \times 2 \times 100}{416} = 5.769 \text{ mmol or } 5.8 \text{ mmol}$$

Checking the prescription of electrolyte maintenance fluid solutions

(Advanced skill)

Prior to administering the electrolyte maintenance solution, the prescription should be checked:

$$\frac{\text{millimoles prescribed} \times \text{drip rate} \times 24 \div \text{weight}}{\text{volume}} = \text{mmol/kg/day}$$

where:

- millimoles prescribed is the total amount of the electrolyte in the solution;
- volume is the volume of fluid that the electrolytes have been put into (e.g. a 100-ml burette or 500-ml bag);

- drip rate is the hourly rate the maintenance fluid is running at;
- weight is in kilogrammes.

For example: a 12-kg child has been prescribed 80% of daily fluid requirements and has half of this as feed. There is also a morphine infusion being administered at 1 ml/h. It has been prescribed that normal daily requirements of electrolytes (see Table 10.1) are required. The infusion is running at 17.3 ml/h. The label on the burette says that the electrolytes added into the burette totalling 100 ml are:

Potassium	5.8 mmol
Sodium	8.6 mmol
Calcium	2.9 mmol
Chloride	5.8 mmol

Potassium

$$\frac{5.8 \times 17.3 \times 24 \div 12}{100} = 2.0 \text{ mmol/kg/day}$$

Sodium

$$\frac{8.6 \times 17.3 \times 24 \div 12}{100} = 2.97 \text{ mmol/kg/day}$$

Calcium

$$\frac{2.9 \times 17.3 \times 24 \div 12}{100} = 1 \text{ mmol/kg/day}$$

Chloride

$$\frac{5.8 \times 17.3 \times 24 \div 12}{100} = 2.0 \text{ mmol/kg/day}$$

Calculating drug infusions
(Advanced skill)
(1) How much drug to add to a 50-ml syringe to give the correct drug infusion dose where the dose is prescribed in micrograms (mcg) per kilogramme per **hour**:

$$\frac{\frac{\text{Desired dose}}{(\text{in } 1\,\text{ml})} \times \frac{\text{weight}}{(\text{kg})} \times \frac{50}{(\text{ml})}}{1000} = \text{mg (in syringe)}$$

For example: a 10-kg child requires midazolam of 100 mcg/kg/h

$$\frac{100 \times 10 \times 50}{1000} = 50$$

so, add 50 mg to the 50-ml syringe and fill the syringe to 50 ml with fluid (e.g. 5% Dx). Running the infusion at 1 ml/h will give 100 mcg/kg/h.

(2) Checking an existing drug infusion running in micrograms per kilogramme per **hour**:

$$\frac{\frac{\text{mg (in}}{\text{infusion})} \times \frac{\text{rate}}{(\text{ml})} \div \frac{\text{weight}}{(\text{kg})} \times \frac{1000}{(\text{mg to mcg})}}{50\,\text{ml (volume put in the syringe)}} = \text{mcg/kg/h}$$

For example: a 5-kg infant has a morphine infusion running at 1 ml/h and the prescription is 20 mcg/kg/h.

Look at the drug label to determine the amount of drug in the syringe.

$$\frac{5 \times 1 \div 5 \times 1000}{50} = 20\,\text{mcg/kg/h}$$

(3) How much drug to add to a 50-ml syringe to give the correct drug infusion dose where the prescription is in micrograms per kilogramme per **minute**:

$$\frac{\frac{\text{Desired dose}}{(\text{in } 1\text{ ml})} \times \frac{\text{weight}}{(\text{kg})} \times \frac{50}{(\text{ml})} \times \frac{60}{(\text{min})}}{1000} = \text{mg (in syringe)}$$

For example: a 7.5-kg child requires dopamine of 5 mcg/kg/min

$$\frac{5 \times 7.5 \times 50 \times 60}{1000} = 112.5$$

so, add 112 mg to the 50-ml syringe and fill the syringe to 50 ml with fluid (e.g. 5% Dx). Running the infusion at 1 ml/h will give 5 mcg/kg/min.

(4) Checking an existing drug infusion running in micrograms per kilogramme per **minute**:

$$\frac{\text{mg (in infusion)} \times \frac{\text{rate}}{\text{(ml)}} \div \frac{\text{weight}}{\text{(kg)}} \div \frac{60}{\text{(min)}} \times \frac{1000}{\text{(mg to mcg)}}}{50 \text{ ml (volume put in the syringe)}} = \text{mcg/kg/h}$$

For example: a 18-kg child has a salbutamol infusion running at 1 ml/h and the prescription is 2 mcg/kg/min.

Look at the drug label to determine the amount of drug in the syringe

$$\frac{108 \times 1 \div 18 \div 60 \times 1000}{50} = 2 \text{ mcg/kg/min}$$

INDWELLING CATHETER ASSESSMENT
(Basic skill)
When a child has a catheter in situ check the following:

- Child:
  - there is no discharge, odour, redness, pain or swelling at the site of insertion;
  - the urethral entrance has been washed with soap and water regularly as part of normal hygiene (see Chapter 14);
  - supra-pubic insertion sites are cleaned as per local wound policy.
- Catheter:
  - there is no traction on the catheter which can lead to bladder trauma;
  - the catheter is changed according to local policy, e.g. non-silicone catheters should be changed every 7 days.
- Tubing:
  - is anchored to the patient so that there is no traction on the catheter;
  - is laid out so there is no looping and it drains adequately into the measuring chamber;

o the catheter bag is emptied regularly (at the end of each shift);
o and bags are changed according to local policy.

FLUID BALANCE
(Basic skill)
A recording should be made of the child's fluid input and output where this information is required for ongoing clinical decision-making. Further, intravenous fluid and drug administration should be documented according to local policy.

Calculating hourly or 24-hourly balances (e.g. +ve 200 ml or −ve 150 ml) and using this information alone for decision-making is fraught with inaccuracies due to:

- inadequate insensible loss calculation (sweat, fever, temperature warming/cooling device use, bowel patterns, loss/gain through respiration/humidification);
- inaccurate calculation of all losses, e.g. venepuncture, blood sampling, wound loss, urine catheter bypass, vomiting;
- inaccurate calculation of all fluid gains, e.g. drug administration, lipids;
- inaccurate calculation of fluid shifts, e.g. oedema, ascites.

Fluid balance is assessed more accurately by undertaking assessment of:

- hydration status (as above);
- urine specific gravity (a high reading indicates hypovolaemia and a low reading may indicate hypervolaemia)
- weight;
- laboratory tests (advanced skill):
  o acid–base balance (see Chapter 3)
  o urea (a high level may be associated with fluid loss):

> Normal level:
>> Neonate 1.1–4.3 mmol/L (*Normal level in your unit:*)
>> Child 1.8–6.4 mmol/L (*Normal level in your unit:*)

  o creatinine (an increased level may be seen with fluid loss and vice versa)

Normal level:
> Neonate 27–88 mmol/L   (*Normal level in your unit:*)
> Child 27–62 mmol/L   (*Normal level in your unit:*)

- o sodium (a high level may be associated with fluid loss)
- o serum osmolality (an increased level may indicate fluid loss and vice versa)

> Normal level:
> 280–295 mOsm/L   (*Normal level in your unit:*)

- o haematocrit (a high level may indicate fluid loss and vice versa)

> Normal level:
> Neonate 40–60%   (*Normal level in your unit:*)
> Infant 30–45%   (*Normal level in your unit:*)
> Child 30–40%   (*Normal level in your unit:*)

BLOOD GLUCOSE
(Basic skill)

Blood sugar levels (BSL) can be assessed at the bedside following training with the blood glucose device. Children, especially young children and infants, are less able to store glucose and then convert glucose if required. A child with a high BSL can quickly use up his or her glucose and become hypoglycaemic. Frequent bedside point-of-testing monitoring is required.

> Normal level:
> 3–7 mmol/L   (*Normal level in your unit:*)

Check BSL 4–6 hourly if acutely ill but stable and 1–4 hourly if critically ill and unstable. Always recheck levels following any corrective procedure, e.g. extra glucose or insulin. In critically ill children, insulin resistance can develop.

Check for signs of hypoglycaemia:

- pallor
- irritability or jitteryness
- decreased level of consciousness
- sweating

Check for signs of hyperglycaemia:

- decreased level of consciousness
- ketone breath
- dehydration

Case Study

Henry is an 18-month-old 12-kg boy, admitted with diarrhoea and vomiting for 3 days. Your physical examination reveals the following findings: normal temperature, increased respiratory rate (38), normal blood pressure, heart rate 160, pulses slightly weak, capillary refill time 3 seconds, decreased urine output, decreased skin turgor, weak cry (no tears) and slightly lethargic, eyes slightly sunken (according to Mum) and dry mouth.

Moderate dehydration (7%) is diagnosed due to diarrhoea and vomiting.

Approximate deficit calculation = $7 \times 12 \times 10 = 840$ ml
Normal maintenance fluids = $(100 \times 10) + (50 \times 2) = 1100$
Total fluids to be administered over 24 hours = 1940 ml
An IV infusion of dextrose/0.9% saline is set to run at

$$\frac{1940}{24} = 81 \, \text{ml/h}$$

Serum electrolyte results will indicate the requirement for the addition of electrolytes. Oral rehydration fluids are commenced and increased as tolerated, decreasing the IV infusion accordingly.

SUMMARY

Early recognition of fluid and electrolyte imbalances is essential in children and infants. Health care practitioners must use a range of assessment skills to evaluate hydration status in an ongoing manner to prevent cardiorespiratory collapse.

REFERENCES

American Association of Critical Care Nurses (2001) A guide to pediatric fluid replacement and maintenance. *Nursing*, **31** (12), 32.

Gill, D. & O'Brien, N. (2002) *Paediatric Clinical Examination Made Easy*, 4th edn. Churchill Livingston, Edinburgh.

Lam, W.H. (1998) Fluids in paediatric patients. *Care of the Critically Ill*, **14** (3), 93–96.

Lorenz, J.M. (1997) Assessing fluid and electrolyte status in the newborn. *Clinical Chemistry*, **43** (1), 205–210.

O'Callaghan, C. & Stephenson, T. (2002) *Pocket Paediatrics*. Churchill Livingstone, Edinburgh.

Park, M.K. (2002) *Pediatric Cardiology*, 4th edn. Mosby, St. Louis.

Resuscitation Council (UK) (2004) *European Paediatric Life Support Course Provider Manual*. Resuscitation Council (UK), London.

Roberts, K.E. (2001) Fluid and electrolyte regulation. In: Curley, M.A.Q. & Moloney-Harmon, P.A. (eds) *Critical Care Nursing of Infants and Children*, 2nd edn. W.B. Saunders, Philadelphia.

Stack, C. & Dobbs, P. (2004) *Essentials of Paediatric Intensive Care*. Greenwich Medical, London.

Wong, D. (1995) *Whaley and Wong's Nursing Care of Infants and Children*, 5th edn. Mosby, St Louis.

11 | The Head and Neck

Lorrie Lawton

INTRODUCTION

This chapter discusses the examination of the head, eyes, ears, nose and throat (HEENT). It looks at the examination techniques for each age group, offering suggestions and tips to aid your examination. The examination of the HEENT does require the health care practitioner to have an array of skills, which need to be tailored to the child's specific age, growth and development. A variety of examination equipment needs to be mastered to ensure that the child does not become anxious. Therefore to examine the HEENT comprehensively the health care practitioner needs to have a calming and reassuring manner when approaching the child.

LEARNING OBJECTIVES

By the end of this chapter the reader will be able to:

❑ Develop an array of examination techniques for children of all ages.
❑ Understand different approaches required to examine the HEENT.
❑ Be able to assess the cranial nerve function in children.

HISTORY

Specific aspects to enquire about include:

• headaches (use pain scale), associated symptoms, circumstances making them worse or better;

- vision, including changes that were sudden or gradual, circumstances that make it worse or better; how vision is affected, e.g. blurring, specks, flashing;
- use of glasses;
- inflammation or excessive tearing of the eye;
- hearing;
- eye ache;
- vertigo;
- tinnitus;
- history of any ear infections or discharge from the ear;
- any 'colds' or upper respiratory tract infections, sore throat (see Chapter 2);
- problems with teething/caries.

PHYSICAL EXAMINATION OF THE HEAD

The head accounts for one fourth of the body length and one third of the body weight at birth, whereas at full maturity it only accounts for one eighth of the body length and one tenth of the body weight (Bickley 2005). The head should be inspected and palpated for (basic skill):

- shape
- position
- symmetry

The bones of the skull are separated by sutures, which in infants and children are movable joints. The fontanelles are where the major sutures intersect in the anterior and posterior portion of the skull. The anterior fontanelle is diamond shaped, and measures about 4–5 cm at its widest part. It closes by 12–18 months of age. The posterior fontanelle is triangular shaped and measures about 0.5–1 cm at its widest part and it closes by the age of 2 months (Muscari 2001). Noting the age of the child, assess whether or not the fontanelles are still palpable. Delays in closure of the fontanelle may be due to:

- normal variation
- hypothyroidism
- arteriovenous malformation
- hydrocephalus

- rickets
- cretinism
- syphilis (rare) (Gill & O'Brien 1998; Muscari 2001).

Palpate the anterior and posterior fontanelles for size (basic skill). A large fontanelle (greater than 4–5 cm in diameter) may be normal, but it can indicate:

- subdural haematoma
- increased intracranial pressure
- osteogenesis imperfecta
- hypothyrodism
- rickets (Muscari 2001)

Palpate the sutures (advanced skill), which are felt as ridges until about 6 months, and the fontanelles, which feel like soft concavities. Note that:

- intracranial pressure is reflected in the amount of tenseness and fullness seen and felt in the anterior fontanelle;
- increased intracranial pressure produces a bulging anterior fontanelle (see Chapter 7). This is normally seen when the baby cries, coughs or vomits;
- pulsation of the fontanelle reflects the peripheral pulses;
- when palpating the infant's fontanelles for fullness and tension ensure that the infant is settled and ideally being held upright (Bickley 2005).

A bulging fontanelle may be indicative of:

- meningitis
- brain tumour
- lead poisoning
- subdural haematoma
- cardiac failure
- pulmonary insufficiency
- vitamin A excess (Muscari 2001).

A depressed fontanelle may be indicative of:

- dehydration
- malnutrition (Muscari 2001).

Marked pulsation of the fontanelle may be indicative of:

- increased intracranial pressure
- obstruction of venous return from the head
- increased pulse pressure (Muscari 2001).

The presence of a 'third' fontanelle which is located between the anterior and posterior fontanelle is noted in children with Down syndrome.

Palpate the cranial bones in newborn infants (advanced skill); these may overlap at the sutures to a certain degree:

- This is known as molding, and is necessary to allow for passage of the neonate through the birth canal. It will usually settle within 2 days.
- If the infant was born by caesarean section molding will not be present.
- An odd shape in older infants may indicate premature closure of sutures (craniosyntosis); this could be genetic (Muscari 2001).

Measure the head circumference (basic skill) (see Chapter 9), which should be measured at every physical examination for the first 2 years of life:

- This will determine the rate of growth and the size of the head.
- Along with weight and height, this can be charted on growth charts. The size of the head circumference reflects the rate of growth of the cranium and its contents. Note that the rate of growth is great in the first 6 years, starting at 25% of adult size at birth through to 95% of adult size by age 6 (Bukatko & Daehler 1998).
- A large head may indicate macrocephaly, a small head microcephaly.

Inspect the newborn scalp (basic skill); it is often bruised and oedematous around the occipitoparietal region:

- This is a normal finding and is called caput succedaneum and is caused by the drawing of that portion of the scalp into the cervical os when the amniotic sac ruptures. The vacuum caused by the loss of amniotic fluids in utero causes capillaries to distend, leading to bruising and oedema. This will usually settle within the first 24 hours of life.

Inspect the symmetry of the head and face (basic skill):

- Asymmetry of the cranial vault, called plagiocephaly, indicates that the infant is lying on one side all the time. There is flattening of the occiput on the dependent side and a prominence of the frontal region on the opposite side.
- Once the baby becomes more active, this will naturally disappear.

Note that when palpating the infant's skull do not put excessive pressure of the thumb and forefinger over the temporo-parietal or parieto-occipital area. You may feel that the underlying bones give way temporarily, in a ping-pong snapping manner (Muscari 2001). This is know as craniotabs and it may result from increased intracranial pressure (from hydrocephaly, metabolic disorders such as rickets, and from infection such as congenital syphilis) (Bickley 2005). *Purposeful elicitation of this finding is not recommended.*

If raised intracranial pressure is suspected, percussing (see Chapter 1 for technique) (advanced skill) the parietal bone on each side by tapping your index or middle finger directly against its surface will produce a 'cracked pot' sound. This is known as MacEwen's sign, and is normal in infants prior to closure of their cranial sutures. However, it can be seen in older infants and children who have increased intracranial pressure that causes closed cranial sutures to separate, e.g. in brain tumour (Muscari 2001; Bickley 2005).

Listen to both sides of the skull for the bruit of an intracranial arteriovenous malformation in infants (advanced skill); it is continuous and loud and may cause heart failure. A quiet systolic bruit over the anterior fontanelle is normal in infants.

Inspect for symmetry and normal movements of the face (basic skill). Table 11.1 shows facial features and causes.

Assess the colour, texture and distribution of the child's hair (basic skill). Scalp hair is normally:

- lustrous
- silky

Table 11.1 Facial features associated with specific conditions/syndromes.
(Adapted from Muscari 2001.)

Condition/syndrome	Facial features
Fetal alcohol syndrome	Short palpebral fissures Wide and flattened philtrum Thin lips
Congenital syphilis	Bulging of the frontal bones Nasal bridge depression (saddle nose) Inflammation and fissuring of the mouth and lips
Congenital hypothyroidism	Low-set hair line Sparse eyebrows Enlarged tongue
Facial nerve palsy	Nasolabial fold on the affected side is flattened Paralysis of the facial nerve Eye does not close Accentuated during crying
Down's syndrome	Small rounded head Hypertelorism Flattened nasal bridge Oblique palpebral fissures Small, low-set ears Relatively large tongue
Hyperthyroidism	'Staring' eyes True exophthalmos rare in children

- strong
- without infestation.

In newborns there may be fine hair called lanugo, which covers the newborn's body for the first few weeks of life. Table 11.2 shows differing hair presentations and their causes.

PHYSICAL EXAMINATION OF THE EYES

- Inspect the eyes (basic skill): they will give you information about the general health of the child. Eyes are generally sparkling and shiny (which indicates a child that is healthy) or dry and sunken (which indicates dehydration – see Chapter 10). Note if the eyes are wide set (hypertelorism) or close set (hypotelorism). You may want to measure the inner canthal

Table 11.2 Differing hair presentations and causes. (Adapted from Muscari 2001.)

Hair presentation	Causes
Increased growth of body hair (hirsutism)	Polycystic ovary disease Cushing's syndrome Adrenal hyperplasia Testicular tumours Ovarian tumours Hyperinsulinism Anabolic steroid abuse
Alopecia	Idiopathic Autoimmune disease Stress Thyroid disease Neoplasms Scalp infections Bullous dermatoses Neglect Hair pulling Skin disease Chemotherapy Caustics Radiation
Dull, dry, brittle hair	Poor nutrition Hypothyroidism Overuse of chemical hair products
Dirty, matted hair	Neglect Depression

(inner corner) distance between the two eyes, which is normally 2.5 cm (Engel 2002).

- Inspect the eyelids (basic skill): are they in proper alignment? They should fall between the upper border of the iris and the upper border of the pupils.
  - The appearance of sclera between the upper lids and the iris may be an indication of hydrocephalus (sunset sign), although this may also be a normal variant (see Chapter 7).
  - A drooping eyelid over the pupil may be a normal variant; however, it could be indicative of paralysis of the oculomotor cranial nerve.

- ○ Inward turning of the eyelid is called entropion, and outward turning is called ectropion.
- ○ Look for any redness, swelling or discharge; this may indicate inflammation of the lacrimal duct from a blocked tear duct.
- ○ Inspecting the newborn's eyes is difficult as the eyes are usually held tight shut. Bright lights cause the newborn to blink; therefore any examination of the eyes should be conducted in subdued lighting (Bickley 2005). Examine the newborn when the baby is upright, and if necessary sucking. The child's eyes usually open in this position (Gill & O'Brien 1998).
- • Inspect the eyebrows (basic skill) for even symmetrical hair growth: they should not meet in the midline.
- • Inspect the conjunctiva (basic skill): if the child is co-operative you can pull the lower lids down as the child looks up. If not you may be able to see the conjunctiva by asking the child to look in different directions.
  - ○ Look for pallor (indicating anaemia) or signs of inflammation (indicating an infection).
- • Inspect the sclera (basic skill): it should be white.
  - ○ Look for any yellowing (indicating jaundice).
- • Inspect the irises (basic skill): they should be round and clear, and may be different colours.
- • Inspect the pupils (basic skill): (see Chapter 7 for the technique of direct and consensual assessment of pupil reactions).
  - ○ Pupils that are equal and react to light may have the finding recorded as PERL × x (x being the number of millimetres the pupil is measured as).
  - ○ In children less than 5 months old, slight pupil inequality is normal. It should not be considered serious unless it is accompanied by other central nervous system findings.
  - ○ Accommodation (the ability of the child's pupils to focus on far and then near objects) is assessed by having the child focus on a light or finger about 40 cm in front of his or her face. Move it in towards the eyes; the pupils should constrict.

Extraocular eye movement (EOEM)
(Advanced skill)

Assessment of the eye movements in an infant can be difficult. However, with patience and practice it is possible.

- Hold the baby upright in your outstretched hands, stabilising the baby's head with your thumbs.
- The practitioner rotates slowly with the baby in one direction.
- The baby should open his or her eyes; the eyes should look in the direction you are turning.
- Stop and the eyes should look in the opposite direction, following a few unsustained nystagmoid movements (Bickley 2005).

There are two tests for strabismus:

(1) The corneal light reflex (Hirschberg test):
   - The child needs to look straight ahead.
   - Shine a light directly into the eyes from a distance of about 40 cm.
   - The light should shine symmetrically into the centre of each cornea.
   - Epicanthal folds may give an impression of misalignments.
   - Intermittent alternating convergent strabismus is normal for the first 6 months of life.
(2) The cover test:
   - Ask the child to look at your nose.
   - Then cover one of the child's eyes.
   - Observe the uncovered eye for any movement.
   - While the child is still focused on your eye, uncover the other eye and observe it for movement; no movement should be noted in either eye when the cover is removed.
   - Infants under the age of 6 months display physiologic strabismus due to poor neuromuscular control of the eye muscles. However, this test may be impossible to complete in this age group.

The cardinal fields of gaze test examines the function of each muscle and nerve supplying and controlling the movement of each eye. Children younger than 2–3 years of age may not be able to cooperate with this test:

- Ask the child to sit still and look forward.
- Ask the child to follow your finger/toy/penlight (whichever you choose to use) with his or her eyes only (not to move the head).
- Move the object and watch the child's eyes as they move in six directions:
  1. left lateral
  2. left lateral superior
  3. left lateral inferior
  4. right lateral
  5. right lateral superior
  6. right lateral inferior
- This can be achieved by moving the object through a wide H shape. Observe for a nystagmus that is easily elicited. A few beats of nystagmus in the far lateral gaze can be normal.

Visual acuity
(Advanced skill)
There is no test that accurately measures visual acuity in children under the age of 3 years. Assessment of the visual acuity in very young children can be assessed grossly by observing their interest in bright objects or a light. Table 11.3 shows normal visual development for different age groups.

In children over the age of 3 years the Snellen E chart is an adequate visual test. When a child is able to articulate letters, a traditional Snellen chart may be used. A pictures chart can also be used if the child is unable to read, or does not speak English (Allen test). The Snellen chart gives a number which indicates the degree of visual acuity when the child is able to read that line of letters at a distance of 6 m. If the child wears glasses the test should be completed using correct vision and then uncorrected vision.

Table 11.3 Normal vision development. (Adapted from Muscari 2001.)

Age	Normal development
Neonate	Visual range 45° Optic nerve and peripheral vision are functional Pupil and corneal reflexes present Central vision not yet developed Near sighted Can briefly follow colourful object Doll's eye reflex
4–6 weeks	Can focus on objects further away
2–3 months	Convergence on near objects – well developed Doll's eye reflex disappears
4–5 months	Able to accommodate to near objects Eye muscles can hold eyes straight
6 months	Can see more clearly at distance Can fix gaze on object
12 months	Can follow rapidly moving objects
18–24 months	Accommodation is well developed Able to fixate on small objects for up to a minute
4–6 years	Depth perception is fully developed by 6 years
7 years	Ocular development is complete

- Place the Snellen chart 6 m from the child.
- Ask the child:
    - to cover one eye with a 'pirate's patch' or other cover;
    - either to point to the direction of the legs of the 'E' on the chart;
    - or to say the letter or the picture;
    - to read to the smallest line possible;
- Three or four correct responses on one line are needed.
- Note the number on this line; this is the top number.
- Repeat the test on the other eye.

To record the visual acuity, the distance from the chart is recorded as the lower number and the line correctly responded to as the top number, e.g. line four at a distance of 6 m is recorded as 'Left eye 4/6, Right eye 4/6'.

Visual fields
(Advanced skill)
This can be performed in children when they are at an age when they can indicate either verbally or behaviourally that they can see the object. Because there is a certain amount of restraint being placed on the child, make this exercise into a game.

- Sit the child on the parent/carer's lap.
- Ask the parent/carer to keep the child's head midline.
- Encourage the child to look directly into your eyes.
- Use a toy or different toys.
- Stand in front of the child and without him or her seeing what the toy is, hold the toys behind the child at a horizontal level to the eyes.
- Slowly bring the toys around to the front of the child in a circling motion at about a distance of 40cm from the head.
- Note when the child can see the toy.
- The child should be able to see both toys at the same time.
- You may have to do one side at a time and make a judgement that the child can see both sides at about the same gaze.
- Repeat coming from a 45° angle from the child's eyes above the ears.
- Repeat coming from a 45° angle from the child's eyes below the ears.

In older children and young people, you may want to use the adult technique of wiggling your fingers as you bring them around and into the field of vision, asking the young person to tell you when he or she sees your 'wiggling fingers'.

Ophthalmoscope examination
(Advanced skill)
To elicit a *red reflex* the practitioner should dim the room and shine a light into the child's eye at a distance of 5cm. There should be a symmetrical bright red glow. No red reflex is called leukocoria and may be caused by:

- cataract
- retinoblastoma
- retinopathy of prematurity (Gill & O'Brien 1998).

In infants and young children, the ophthalmic examination may stop here.

In order to complete a *retinal fundoscopy* patience and practice are required. The room should be darkened. The child either should lie supine on a couch, being held still (particularly the head) by the parent/carer, or, if more cooperative, should sit on a chair or the parent/carer's lap (who may have to hold the head still).

- Use your right hand and right eye for the child's right eye, with the left hand placed on the child's forehead so that when you get close to the child, the ophthalmoscope will rest on your hand rather than the child.
- Use your left hand and left eye for the child's left eye, with the right hand placed on the child's forehead.

The procedure for fundoscopy using an ophthalmoscope is as follows:

- Set the ophthalmoscope at 0 diopters and check the strength of the light by shining it on the back of your hand.
- Tell the child to pick a spot over your shoulder to stare at – this could be a specific picture of a cartoon character on the wall.
- Begin at an angle of 15° and a distance of about 30 cm.
- Shine the light into the child's pupil.
- Locate the red reflex.
- Move slowly towards the child; you will become very close to the child, almost touching the eyelashes.
- When the retina is seen, focus carefully (moving the diopter, usually 0 to –2 in infants) and follow a blood vessel centrally to the optic disc.
- Observe the optic disc for colour (yellow-orange) and shape (round), and identify the physiologic cup; note any oedema (indicating increased intracranial pressure).
- Observe the size of arterioles and veins, checking for nicking at arteriovenous crossings.
- Ask the child to look into the light; examine the macule (not well able to be evaluated without mydriatic eye drops).
- Repeat the procedure with the other eye.

Occasionally a mydriatic eye drop can be used to facilitate examination. This is mainly completed by ophthalmic specialists.

PHYSICAL EXAMINATION OF THE EARS
Inspection and palpation
(Basic skill)

- Draw an imaginary horizontal line from the corner of the eye towards the back of the head; the top of the ear should just meet or cross this line.
- A small, deformed or low-set auricle may indicate associated congenital defects (Bickley 2005).
- Palpate the auricle, noting tenderness or lesions.
- The pinna should be in a perpendicular line to the rest of the ear or at no more than 10° deviance (Engel 2002).
- Inspect the external ear for discharge, swelling or redness. The presence of soft yellow-brown ear wax is normal; the absence of wax may indicate over-vigorous cleaning.
  - Foul-smelling yellow or green discharge may indicate ruptured tympanic membrane.
  - Bloody discharge may indicate trauma, foreign body or ruptured tympanic membrane.
  - Clear discharge may indicate a cerebral spinal fluid leak and a fractured skull.
- Palpate the mastoid prominence for tenderness; this may indicate mastoiditis.

Hearing acuity
(Advanced skill)

Hearing loss is the most common disability. Hearing is normally fully developed at birth; however, the neural pathways that enable the child to interpret the sound are still being developed.

Normal hearing for children by age is as follows:

- 2–3 months: the infant can turn the head to the side of the sound.
- 4–6 months: the infant can localize sounds made below the ear, followed by sounds made above the ear.

- 6–8 months: the infant can localize sounds by turning the head in a curving arc.
- 8–10 months: the infant can localize sounds by turning the head diagonally and directly towards the sound.
- 10–12 months: the child can control and adjust his or her own response to sound.
- 3–4 years: hearing reaches maturity.
- 13 years: auditory acuity reaches its peak.

Infants

Hearing in this age group can be assessed by using the acoustic blink reflex (Bickley 2005). The test is crude at best, and it is not a diagnostic test for deafness. The following is a positive response:

- Stand behind the child.
- At approximately 30 cm from the child, produce a sharp sound such as snapping fingers or clapping hands.
- The child should blink.

Pre-schooler

It is important for the practitioner to assume that the parent's assessment of the child's hearing loss is accurate unless it is proven otherwise. A quick assessment can be made as follows:

- Stand 0.5–1 m in front of the child.
- Give a command such as 'Can you give me the teddy please?'.

School age/young person

- Stand 0.3 m behind the child.
- Ask the child to cover one ear.
- Whisper three numbers in random order.
- Ask the child to repeat what you have said.
- Repeat with the other ear.

Otoscope examination

(Advanced skill)

The next step is to complete an internal examination of the ear using an otoscope. The practitioner needs patience and practice in order to successfully complete this examination on a child. It should be the last part of your assessment of the ears, as it can be frightening for the child to have an otoscope placed in the ear. Initially the practitioner needs to gain the co-operation of both the child and the parent. Allowing the child to hold and play with the otoscope will reassure the child. Also demonstrating what you are about to do on a toy will allow the child to relax. The procedure for the use of the otoscope is as follows:

- Ensure correct position of the child – either supine or on the parent's lap:
  - ○ Supine: ask the parent to hold the child's arms extended and close to the side of the head, therefore limiting movement from side to side.
  - ○ On parent's lap: sit the child sideways, with one arm tucked behind the parent's back. The parent then holds one of his or her hands across the child's head and forehead against the chest. The other hand holds the child's body still. When the other ear needs to be examined the child needs to be turned around the other way.
- Choose the largest speculum that fits comfortably into the ear canal.
- Hold the otoscope like a pen; this allows for sudden movement of the child's head. You may also like to place your third, fourth and fifth fingers on the child's head so that your hand will go with the child's head if it moves.
- Straighten the ear canal:
  - ○ children less than 3 years: pull the earlobe gently down and out;
  - ○ children older than 3 years: pull the pinna up and back.
- Gently insert the otoscope into the ear canal; observe for any redness, trauma or discharge
- Locate the tympanic membrane.
- Observe the tympanic membrane for a cone of light, bony landmarks, colour, any bulging or holes.

Note that:

- any pain on movement of the pinna may indicate otitis media or otitis externa;

- pain on insertion of the otoscope into the ear canal will also indicate otitis externa or presence of a foreign body;
- a red bulging tympanic membrane is indicative of otitis media.

Pre-school children often place small foreign bodies in their ears. These could be small toys, beads, bits of paper, etc. The removal of these foreign bodies can be a challenge to any practitioner:

- Examine the ear by using the otoscope.
- If the foreign body is easily reached within the ear canal then removal may be possible using a pair of forceps.
- Care needs to be taken not to push the foreign body further down the ear canal and perforate the tympanic membrane.
- Occasionally the practitioner can use the tip of a Yankeur suction tube to suck the foreign body out.
- If the practitioner is unable to remove the foreign body or the child becomes too distressed and uncooperative then a referral to an ENT (ear, nose and throat) specialist is necessary.

PHYSICAL EXAMINATION OF THE NOSE
Inspection
(Basic skill)
The nose should be observed for:

- symmetry
- deformity
- bruising
- wounds
- epistaxis

A flat nasal bridge in infants is normal; however, it is also notable in Downs syndrome.

Nare patency
(Advanced skill)
Neonates are obligatory nasal breathers; therefore any obstruction of the nose can lead to hypoxia and apnoea (see Chapter 2).

To assess patency in the neonate:

- Palpate the movement of air in each nostril with your fingers; place the tip of your finger near the nare outlet.
- Listen to the sound of air by the nare with a stethoscope.
- Note condensation on a mirror held over the anterior nares.
- If there is a suspicion of an obstruction, then a catheter can be passed through each nostril into the posterior nasopharynx.

To assess patency in the older child:

- Occlude one nostril with your finger and ask the child to sniff.
- Repeat with the other nostril.

Sinuses
(Basic skill)
Palpate the sinuses in the child 8 years and over (too small in younger children) by gently pressing over the sinus locations and asking if the child feels any pain or demonstrates a painful response.

- The ethmoid and maxillary sinuses are present at birth.
- The frontal sinus develops around the age of 7 years.
- The sphenoid sinus develops in adolescence (Engel 2002).

Pain or tenderness could indicate sinusitis.

Internal examination
(Advanced skill)
In young children:

- Tilt the head backwards.
- Gently push the nose upward to visualise the internal nasal cavity.
- Use a pen torch to observe the nasal mucosa for colour and consistency.

In older children:

- You can use an otoscope.
- Hold the child as discussed early in examination of the ear.

- Use the largest speculum possible.
- Gently insert the otoscope into the nose.
- Observe the mucosa and the inferior and middle turbinates for colour, swelling, exudates and polyps.

Sense of smell
(Advanced skill)
Sense of smell is poorly developed in the neonate and is difficult to assess. In older children you can make a game of this procedure.

- Ask the child to close eyes.
- Obstruct one of the nostrils.
- Pass a smell (pleasant!) under the nose (the smell used needs to be easily identifiable to the child).
- Ask the child to identify the smell.
- Repeat with the other nostril, using a different scent.

As with ears, the nose is a common receptacle for foreign bodies. If the health care practitioner can easily see the foreign body and it is anterior, removal can be attempted with forceps or a suction catheter. If the foreign body is posterior in the nasal cavity referral to an ENT specialist will be necessary.

Due to the position there is an increased risk of airway obstruction. Another method of removal is known as the 'mother's kiss'. This involves the parent blowing in the child's mouth whilst obstructing the nostril that does not have the foreign body in. The pressure of the parent's 'kiss' forces the foreign body out of the nose.

PHYSICAL EXAMINATION OF THE MOUTH AND THROAT
Do not attempt any examination of the throat if epiglottitis is suspected. By accidentally invoking the gag reflex during the examination you could produce complete laryngeal obstruction. Keep the child sitting up and call for anaesthetic assistance.

Inspection
(Basic skill)
The mouth (see Chapter 14) and throat should be inspected for:

- healthy, pink buccal cavity;
- status of tooth development:
  - deciduous teeth come through from 6 months (central incisors) to 2 years (upper second molar);
  - permanent teeth come through from 6 years (central incisors and first molars) to 13 years (premolars and second molars) and late adolescence/early adulthood (third molars or 'wisdom' teeth) (Chamley 2005);
- size and presence of tonsils: in both early and late childhood the tonsils are relatively larger than in infancy and adolescence. A white exudate on the tonsils suggests *streptococcal tonsillitis*, a thick grey adherent exudate suggests *diptheritic tonsillitis*, and necrosis suggests *infectious mononucleosis* (Bickley 2005).

To inspect the mouth and pharynx of a newborn:

- lie the baby supine;
- use a tongue blade and torch.

To examine the mouth and pharynx of a child can be difficult.

- Most children are more than willing to open their mouths and say 'ahh'. If the practitioner is quick then all the information that he/she needs can be obtained.
- If the child is reluctant to open the mouth, a direct approach to the front teeth will usually end in failure. You may want to:
  - try again after a few minutes;
  - try the following method if it is necessary to see the throat:
    - It involves inducing the gag reflex, and consequently the parent should be warned.
    - Sit the child on the parent's lap and ask him or her to secure the child's head.
    - Gently push a tongue depressor through the clamped lips, along the buccal mucosa and between the gums and the molars.
    - The child will gag and therefore open the mouth, producing a quick view of the mouth and pharynx (Bickley 2005).

– This should only be done when all other attempts have failed.

Trachea

The trachea should be inspected and palpated (see Chapter 1).

Thyroid gland

(Advanced skill)

The thyroid gland is not visible or palpable in the infant. In the young and older children, ask them to tip their head back and observe for any swelling below the cricoid cartilage. In older children and young people, you may want to stand behind them and palpate the gland with the tips of your fingers. Ask them to swallow and you may be able to feel the isthmus rising. Examination of the thyroid gland is difficult where the patient has a short neck, and therefore not routinely performed in children.

Lymph glands

(Advanced skill)

The neck glands are readily seen in thin children. Normal glands in children are small pea-sized, discrete and non-tender (Gill & O'Brien 1998). As with any examination, the practitioner needs to be logical whilst palpating the lymphatic system. The following outlines one systematic order in which to palpate the lymph glands:

- occipital
- posterior auricular
- pre-auricular
- tonsillar
- submandibular
- submental
- superficial cervical
- posterior cervical
- deep cervical chain
- supraclavicular

Note that:

- The neck glands should be examined from both in front and behind the child.
- The site, size, consistency, tenderness, mobility and attachments of the lymph nodes should be evaluated.
- Lymph nodes are usually non-palpable in infants and young people.
- 'Shotty' nodes which are palpable, small, non-tender and mobile, are common between the ages of 3 and 12 years (Muscari 2001).

Cranial nerves

(Advanced skill)

The cranial nerves are part of the neurological system. However, examination of the cranial nerves often takes place during examination of the head and neck. Examination of cranial nerves in children can be a great challenge to the health care practitioner. As with all examinations, practitioners may need to adapt what they would normally do for adults to the child. There are 12 cranial nerves that each need to be tested in a logical and systematic way to ensure that no abnormality is detected. These 12 cranial nerves and their basic functions are outlined in Table 11.4. Note that a commonly used ditty has been included; some health care practitioners find this useful for remembering all the cranial nerves. *Write your own in if you have another.*

Examination of the cranial nerves of a co-operative child or young person is the same as that for an adult, and is outlined in Table 11.5. Health care practitioners may need to adapt how they ask children to do some of the tests and make it fun for them, as they are then more likely to co-operate. If the child is uncooperative or an infant, then you will need to make some decisions about the cranial nerves whilst watching the child, e.g. the normal movement of the eye can be assessed whilst watching a child playing. Table 11.6 outlines differing examination techniques for the pre-schooler and Table 11.7 for the infant. Within the clinical setting, cranial nerve I (olfactory) is rarely tested. However, if the child reports any changes in sense of

Table 11.4 The cranial nerves. (Abbreviations: *EOEM* extraocular eye movement; *M* motor; *S* sensory; *ant* anterior; *post* posterior.)

A commonly used ditty (write in your own if you like)	Number	Name	Function
On	I	Olfactory	Sense of smell
Old	II	Optic	Vision
Olympus	III	Oculomotor	Pupil constriction, eye opening, most EOEM
Towering	IV	Trochlear	EOEM (downwards and inwards movements)
Tops	V	Trigeminal	(M) Temporal and masseter muscle contraction (S) Ophthalmic, maxillary and mandibular
A	VI	Abducens	EOEM (lateral deviation)
Farmer	VII	Facial	(M) Facial movements, closing eyes, closing mouth (S) Taste (salt, etc.) on ant two-thirds of tongue
And	VIII	Auditory	Hearing and balance
Gardener	IX	Glossopharyngeal	(M) Pharynx, tongue (S) Post portions of eardrum and ear canal, the pharynx and post tongue (including taste)
Viewed	X	Vagus	(M) Palate, pharynx, larynx (S) Pharynx and larynx
Some	XI	Spinal accessory	(M) Sternomastoid and upper portions of trapezius
Hops	XII	Hypoglossal	(M) Tongue movement

Table 11.5 Older child/young person cranial nerve testing. (Readers are invited to add their own comments in each of the boxes.)

Cranial nerve	The test (add others you may use)
I	Check nare patency (as above)
II	Visual acuity (Snellen chart) (as above) Visual fields (as above) Pupil reactions (as above) Accommodation (as above) Ocular fundi (as above)
II–III	EOEM (most) (as above) Pupil reactions (as above) Eye opening
IV	EOEM (downward and inward movement) (as above)
V	(M) Place fingers on the temporal and masseter muscles and ask young person to clench his/her teeth; note the strength of the muscles during contraction (S) Explain procedure to young person first Part 1 • Ask young person to close eyes • Use sharp yet safe object with a blunt end • Test the lateral forehead, cheek and lateral jaw (ophthalmic, maxillary, mandibular) for a 'sharp' or 'dull' sensation (apply both in no recognisable order) to compare sides Part 2 • Ask young person to close eyes • Ask him/her to say when he/she feels the application • Use a fine wisp of cotton wool to dab on the face, testing the ophthalmic, maxillary, mandibular areas as above
VI	EOEM (lateral deviation) (as above)
VII	(M) Note any asymmetry in facial expressions; ask young person to raise eyebrows, frown, close eyes very tightly, smile, puff out cheeks (S) Not usually tested
VIII	Hearing acuity (as above)
IX	(M) Have young person stick out tongue all the way or say 'ahh'; observe movement of uvula and soft palate (should rise) Test gag (only if necessary) (S) Not usually tested
X	(M) Palate, pharynx, larynx; is the voice normal? is there any difficulty swallowing? (S) Pharynx and larynx
XI	Place your hand on the side of the young person's face and have him/her push your hand away with his/her head; test both sides Ask young person to shrug shoulders while you push down with your hands to see how strong you are
XII	Have young person stick out tongue all the way and note symmetry

Table 11.6 Pre-schooler cranial nerve testing. (Readers are invited to add their own comments in each of the boxes.)

Cranial nerve	The test (add others you may use)
I	Difficult to test
II	Visual acuity (Snellen E chart or Allen test) (as above) Pupil reactions (as above) Visual fields (parents holding head) (as above)
III, IV, VI	Use toy and note tracking; parent may have to hold head (as above)
V	(M) Have child clench teeth, chew or swallow food (S) Game with soft cotton wool (see Table 11.5)
VII	Have the child make faces or imitate you (including moving your eyebrows); observe symmetry and facial movements
VIII	Hearing acuity (as above)
IX–X	Have child stick whole tongue out or say 'ahh'; observe movement of uvula and soft palate Test gag (if necessary)
XI	Have child push your hand away with his/her head Have child shrug shoulders while you push down with your hands to see how strong you are
XII	Have child stick out tongue all the way and note symmetry

smell then this needs to be tested. Each health care practitioner needs to find his or her own way to test the cranial nerves; however, you must ensure that all the cranial nerves are tested.

DOCUMENTATION

Table 11.8 shows a summary of techniques and documentary findings for each age group.

SUMMARY

Examination of the head, eyes, ears, nose and throat is common for all health care practitioners. Although the actual examina-

Table 11.7 Infant cranial nerve testing. (Readers are invited to add their own comments in each of the boxes.)

Cranial nerve	The test (add others you may use)
I	Difficult to test
II	Have baby regard your face and look for facial response and tracking of bright toy
II–III	In dark room raise baby to sitting position to open eyes, and use light to test for red reflex Assess pupil responses
III, IV, VI	Observe tracking as baby regards your smiling face moving side-to-side
V	(M) Test rooting reflex (see Table 6.9) Test sucking reflex (breast, bottle, pacifier) (see Table 6.9)
VII	Observe baby crying and smiling Note symmetry of face and forehead
VIII	Test acoustic blink reflex (blinking of both eyes in response to sound) Observe tracking in response to sound
IX–X	Swallow: observe co-ordination during swallowing Gag: test gag (only if absolutely necessary)
XI	Observe symmetry of shoulders
XII	Observe co-ordination of swallowing, sucking and tongue thrusting Pinch nostrils, observe reflex opening of mouth and note the tip of tongue at midline

tion of this system is the same as for adults, due to the nature of the examination the health care practitioner will need to adapt some of the assessment, taking into account the age, developmental stage and co-operation of the child. However, with patience and practice all practitioners should be successful in the examination of this system. Different aspects of the examination will be needed with different patients and the health care practitioner will need to make clinical decisions on which are needed.

Table 11.8 Summary of techniques and documentary findings for each age group.

Infant

Inspect and palpate the head and hair
Palpate fontanelles and sutures
Inspect scalp and observe any molding in the neonate
Observe symmetry of head and face
Observe for normal facial movements
Auscultate for intra-cranial bruit
Measure head circumference
Inspect eyes, eyelids, eyebrows, conjunctiva, sclera, iris, pupils (direct and consensual reactions as well as accommodation)
Test for strabismus
Test for visual acuity (crude)
Carry out ophthalmoscope examination: red reflexes
Inspect ears for position, inflammation, discharge
Palpate ears for tenderness
Test hearing acuity
Carry out otoscope examination
Inspect nose for symmetry, deformity, bruising, wounds, epistaxis
Assess nare patency
Palpate sinuses
Inspect mouth and pharynx including buccal cavity and dentition
Palpate lymph glands
Test cranial nerves

Normal findings in a 6-month-old

Head: normal shape, symmetrical, sutures just palpable, anterior fontanelle open 2 cm, neither sunken nor bulging, posterior closed; head circumference 44 cm; face symmetrical with normal movements and expressions; light head of hair with slight balding over the occiput; no intracranial bruit
Eyes: bright, conjunctiva pink, sclera white; PERL × 4; a few unsustained nystagmoid movements in left eye; appears to follow coloured objects; blink reflex positive; red reflexes present
Ears: ear canals clear, tympanic membrane with no inflammation; appears to respond to and turn towards sounds
Nose: nasal passages clear, no sinus tenderness
Mouth: clean and pink; no pharyngeal inflammation; no teeth
No lymph glands palpable
Cranial nerves II–XII intact

Pre-schooler

Inspect and palpate the head and hair
Observe symmetry of head and face
Observe for normal facial movements
Measure head circumference (up to 2 years of age)

Table 11.8 *Continued.*

Inspect eyes, eyelids, eyebrows, conjunctiva, sclera, iris, pupils (direct and
  consensual reactions as well as accommodation)
Test for strabismus, attempt cardinal fields of gaze
Test visual acuity
Test visual fields
Carry out ophthalmoscope examination: red reflexes and fundoscopy
Inspect ears for position, inflammation, discharge
Palpate ears for tenderness
Test hearing acuity
Carry out otoscope examination
Inspect nose for symmetry, deformity, bruising, wounds, epistaxis
Assess nare patency
Inspect internal nose
Palpate sinuses
Attempt sense of smell
Inspect mouth and pharynx including buccal cavity and dentition
Palpate lymph glands
Inspect and palpate trachea
Inspect thyroid gland
Test cranial nerves

Normal findings in a 3-year-old
Head: normal shape, symmetrical, no fontanelles palpated; face symmetrical
  with normal movements and expressions; shiny, clean, lustrous hair kept
  short
Eyes: bright, conjunctiva pink, sclera white; PERL × 4; corneal light reflex
  negative; visual acuity R 6/6 L 6/6 with Snellen E chart; red reflexes present
  – fundoscopy not performed
Ears: ear canals clear, tympanic membrane has no inflammation; good cone of
  light; acuity good to voice request
Nose: nasal passages clear, mucosa pink, septum midline
No sinus tenderness
Mouth: clean and pink; no pharyngeal inflammation; deciduous teeth present
No lymph glands palpable
Cranial nerves II–XII intact

Older child/young person
Inspect and palpate the head and hair
Observe symmetry of head and face
Observe for normal facial movements
Inspect eyes, eyelids, eyebrows, conjunctiva, sclera, iris, pupils (direct and
  consensual reactions as well as accommodation)
Test for strabismus, cardinal fields of gaze
Test visual acuity
Test visual fields
Carry out ophthalmoscope examination: red reflexes and fundoscopy

Continued

Table 11.8 *Continued.*

Inspect ears for position, inflammation, discharge
Palpate ears for tenderness
Test hearing acuity
Carry out otoscope examination
Inspect nose for symmetry, deformity, bruising, wounds, epistaxis
Assess nare patency
Inspect internal nose
Palpate sinuses
Assess sense of smell
Inspect mouth and pharynx including buccal cavity and dentition
Palpate lymph glands
Inspect and palpate trachea
Inspect and palpate thyroid gland
Test cranial nerves

Normal findings in a 14-year-old

Head: normal shape, symmetrical; face symmetrical with normal movements
 and expressions; shiny, clean, lustrous hair kept shoulder length
Eyes: bright, conjunctiva pink, sclera white; PERL × 4; extraocular movements
 intact; visual acuity R 6/6 L 6/6 with Snellen E chart; red reflexes present –
 fundoscopy; disc margins sharp
Ears: R ear canal some wax partially obscures tympanic membrane; L ear
 clear, tympanic membrane no inflammation; good cone of light; acuity good to
 whispered voice
Nose: nasal passages clear, mucosa pink, septum midline
No sinus tenderness
Mouth: clean and pink; no pharyngeal inflammation; dentition good – permanent
 teeth intact
No lymph glands palpable
Trachea midline
Thyroid isthmus not palpable
Cranial nerves II–XII intact

REFERENCES

Bickley, L. (2005) *Bate's Guide to Physical Examination and History Taking*, 9th edn. Lippincott, New York.

Bukatko, D. & Daehler, M.W. (1998) *Child Development: A Thematic Approach*, 3rd edn. Houghton Mifflin, Boston.

Chamley, C.A. (2005) Dentition. In: Chamley, C.A., Carson, P., Randall, D. & Sandwell, M. (eds) (2005) *Developmental Anatomy and Physiology of Children: A Practical Approach*. Elsevier, Edinburgh.

Engel, J. (2002) *Mosby's Pediatric Assessment*, 4th edn. Mosby, New York.

Gill, D. & O'Brien, N. (1998) *Paediatric Clinical Examination*, 3rd edn. Churchill Livingstone, London.

Muscari, M. (2001) *Advanced Pediatric Clinical Assessment: Skills and Procedures*. Lippincott, New York.

12 | The Musculoskeletal System

Lorrie Lawton

INTRODUCTION

Musculoskeletal problems are common presenting symptoms in children and young people. They are usually self-limiting in origin but can be a presenting feature of severe, even life-threatening events (Kay *et al*. 2003). Therefore, it is essential that there is a clear and accurate assessment of the child that presents with a musculoskeletal problem. To make an accurate diagnosis the practitioner must take an accurate history, complete a thorough and systemic examination and instigate appropriate investigations.

LEARNING OBJECTIVES

By the end of this chapter the reader will be able to:

❑ Develop history-taking skills in musculoskeletal examination.
❑ Evaluate the musculoskeletal system using a 'look, feel, move' framework.
❑ Understand neurovascular assessment.

HISTORY TAKING

Taking a history from a child with a musculoskeletal injury can be a challenge for any practitioner; however, it is the cornerstone of paediatric problem solving (Gill & O'Brien 1998). It is essential that a clear and concise history be obtained, as this will aid the practitioner in making a clear diagnosis. Children can present with a non-traumatic or traumatic history. Each of these presentations will have a different focus for the history.

History taking in the injured child

Approaching children that are injured can be difficult for a practitioner. If a child is in pain then he/she may be unwilling/unable to give an accurate history. This will also be dependent upon the age of the child and the child's ability to give his or her own history. History may have to be obtained from the parent/carer or individual who was with the child at the time of injury. Therefore, the history obtained may be second or third hand. The health care practitioner must make every effort to try to obtain as accurate a history as possible.

Assessment of the child's pain and treatment is essential if an accurate history is to be obtained. When a child presents with an injury it is essential, along with the history, that the exact mechanism of injury is determined. It is helpful to have a mental picture of the direction, magnitude and duration of the forces applied to the injured part (Wardrope & English 1998). This will aid in the diagnosis of the problem. Again this can be difficult to obtain if the child is unable to describe the exact mechanism of injury or if the injury was not witnessed. Therefore, occasionally the health care practitioner will need to make some assumptions about the exact mechanism of injury. Table 12.1 illustrates some common mechanisms of injury and the common related injuries.

The complete and accurate circumstance surrounding the injury is essential to discover. Some basic questions include:

- What was the date and time of the injury and when was it first noticed?
- Where did the injury occur?
- Who witnessed the injury?
- What was happening before the injury occurred?
- What did the child do after the injury?
- What did the parent/carer do after the injury?
- How long after the injury did the parent/carer wait until seeking care for the child?

(Giardino 2006)

Table 12.1 Mechanism of injury relating to common injuries.

Common injury	Mechanism of injury
Fall onto outstretched hand	Greenstick fractures distal radius and ulna Supracondylar fracture Fractured clavicle Fractured humerus Scaphoid fracture (rare in the under 12s)
Twisting action	Salter Harris fractures fingers
Direct blow to elbow	Radial head fractures Supracondylar fractures Olecranon fractures
Axial traction	Pulled elbow
Inversion injury	Fractured lateral or medial alleles Fractured tibia or fibula
Landing directly on feet	Fractured calcaneum

History taking in the non-injured child
(Basic skill)

Assessment of a child presenting with a non-traumatic musculo-skeletal problem can take considerable amount of time. The history that the practitioner needs to obtain is slightly different:

- The age of the child: some conditions are specifically related to age; for example, irritable hip is more common in children less than 7 years old, and slipped femoral epiphysis usually occurs in young people (Morton & Phillips 1992).
- History of recent illness: some conditions are related to previous viral illness; for example, irritable hip is thought to follow a viral infection 2–3 weeks previously.
- Sequence of events: when did the condition start? Is the condition of slow or rapid onset?

History taking in the child with a suspected non-accidental injury (NAI)
(Advanced skill)

Evidence of abuse can present in a great variety of ways but most commonly as unexplained bruising or fractures (Glasgow

& Graham 1997). It is essential that with any child presenting with a musculoskeletal injury the health care practitioner is clear about the history relating to that injury. However, as discussed earlier, this can be difficult to achieve. Crucial diagnostic clues should not be overlooked, such as:

- incongruity between the (parental) history and the physical signs;
- lack of parental concern or an uncaring attitude towards the child;
- delay in seeking medical attention;
- child looks undernourished (see Chapter 9) and ill-cared for;
- parents describe minor trauma, but the child displays major injury on examination;
- no history of trauma is given (so-called magical injuries);
- injury is described as self-inflicted and is not compatible with the age or developmental abilities of the child;
- serious injury is blamed on younger siblings/playmates;
- parents frequently change General Practitioners or Emergency Departments.

(Giardino 2006)

From the history, if there is any suspicion that the child may be being subjected to abuse, then a careful and thorough examination needs to be completed *following local polices*.

PHYSICAL ASSESSMENT

The assessment of the musculoskeletal system should be systematic and logical; this will ensure that no vital information is missed. The examination of an injured child should obtain the maximum amount of information with a minimum of fuss or distress (Glasgow & Graham 1997). It consists of:

- examining the joint above and below;
- looking, feeling and moving that joint;
- examining the neurovascular function.

Always try to examine the child in an environment that is well lit and relaxed. If the child is young, carry out the examination whilst the child is sitting on the parent/carer's lap. Always remove enough clothing to allow for good examination without compromising the child's privacy and dignity.

Examination of the joint above and below

It is always good practice to examine the joint proximal and distal to the injury, e.g. if the child presents with an injured elbow, then the shoulder and wrist joints must also be examined. This serves two functions:

(1) It provides an opportunity to make contact with the child without causing pain. This will reassure the child and allow confidence to grow, helping to build a good rapport between the child and the practitioner (Wardrope & English 1998).
(2) It will determine other injuries that would have otherwise been missed, e.g. a fracture to the fibula head associated with fractures of the lateral alleles.

Look

(Basic skill)

The initial part of any assessment is to observe the child; watching them walk or play can give a lot of information regarding the child, e.g. the child holding the arm down by his or her side may be indicative of a pulled elbow.

Observing the child's gait assesses if the child is weight bearing or walking with a limp. The normal toddler frequently has a mildly bow-legged gait; this then converts to a knock-kneed posture in the pre-school-aged child (Gill & O'Brien 1998). This is normal and should not cause any concern unless extreme. Table 12.2 illustrates the multiple causes of an acute limp in children (Gill & O'Brien 1998).

Swelling

Observe for:

- swelling or effusion
- deformity
- wounds
- bruising

Table 12.2 Causes of limping in a child.

Irritable hip
Transient synovitis
Pyogenic arthritis
Osteomyelitis
Discitis
Osteochondritis
Puncture wound/verruca/foreign body in foot
Spiral fracture of tibia or fibula
Rheumatoid arthritis
Bone tumour
Trauma
Perthes' disease
Slipped femoral epiphysis
Anaphylactoid purpura
Lymphatic leukaemia
Coagulation disorder
Inguinal hernia
Testicular torsion

Within the joint observe for:

- loss of usual bony landmarks and joint contours
- associated muscle wasting

This could indicate synovial thickening or joint effusion or both (Gill & O'Brien 1998). Effusions are common in injuries of the knee and elbow. Within the elbow joint, acute haemarthrosis will displace the fat pads of the joint. These are seen on the lateral radiographs (must be a true lateral projection).

In the elbow, the fat pad overlies the capsule in the coronoid fossa anteriorly, and lies within the olecranon fossa posteriorly. With a large effusion, the fat pad is narrowed and bulges forward. In children under 2 years, the fat pad may be obliterated and therefore not visible.

Raised fat pad sign may be the only radiographic sign of a fracture. However, fat pads may be seen when there is no fracture present (Thornton & Gyll 1999). Within the knee joint, the presence of a fat/fluid level (lipohaemarthrosis) on radiographs indicates that a fracture is present even if there is no fracture line visible (Thornton & Gyll 1999).

In children there may be more subtle signs even with significant injuries, e.g. in spiral fractures of the tibia there may be only slight swelling and slight pain on palpation (Wardrope & English 1998). Greenstick fractures are notoriously difficult to diagnose clinically and are only confirmed on radiographs. This is due to lack of clinical signs such as swelling, bruising or deformity; the child may only present with 'not using arm'. Therefore, the health care practitioner must not rely on the clinical sign of swelling as an indication of the seriousness of the underlying condition or injury.

Deformity
When observing the limb, it is essential to observe for any deformity.

- Any limb where a deformity is present must be compared with the non-injured limb. Fractures of the radius and ulna, common in school-aged children, can present with gross deformity of the forearm. Also, supracondylar fractures, which make up approximately half of all injuries in the elbow, can present with gross deformity around the elbow. These injuries are common in children aged 4–8 years.
- Joint dislocations are rare in children; however, dislocations of the elbow and the thumb do occur. Shoulder dislocations are only common in teenagers (Thornton & Gyll 1999). If there is obvious deformity of the limb it is essential that the limb is not moved, as this will cause an increased amount of pain and distress for the child. However, it is essential to determine whether there is any wound present over the deformity or if there is any blanching or tenting of the skin over the fracture site.
- The neurovascular status of the limb must also be assessed distally to the injury. This is discussed further later in the text.

Bruising
Bruising over bony prominence is common in childhood. Note the amount of bruising and the age of the bruises. However, patterns of bruising that raise the concern of possible abuse include:

- involvement of multiple areas of the body beyond bony prominences;
- bruises at many stages of healing;
- bruises in non-ambulatory child;
- marking resembling objects, grab marks or slap marks

(Giardino 2006).

There are some differential diagnoses to bruising other than NAI. These include:

- Mongolian spots
- haemangioma
- eczema
- phytophotodermatitis
- erythema multiforme
- idiopathic thrombocytopenic purpura (ITP)

(Giardino 2006).

Wounds

Any wounds that are present should be observed for:

- location (exactly where they are);
- direction (in which way do they progress?);
- shape;
- size: including length, width and depth;
- evidence of underlying bony injury (Guly 1996).

Wounds caused by a blunt force may harbour a fracture of the underlying bone, e.g. a finger trapped in car doors will present with a wound to the pulp and the nail bed and radiographs may indicate an underlying fracture to the distal phalanx (known as tuft fracture). Note that the presence of an underlying fracture will change the management of the wound as it is communicating with a fracture site; the practitioner may need to consider the use of antibiotic therapy to reduce the risk of infection.

In teenagers (12–16 years) a common injury is fracture of the fifth metacarpal, known as a boxer's fracture. The mechanism of injury is a punch with a closed fist. If a child presents with this injury and a laceration is present it must be noted that the lacerated part may have been caused by the teeth of the person who received the punch. If this is present, ensure that there is no fragment of the tooth in the wound (this will be seen on radiograph). Due to the nature of the wound the child should receive antibiotic cover for potential infection.

Once a thorough visual examination of the limb has been completed only then can the practitioner continue with the rest of the examination. If the practitioner does not take time to thoroughly observe the limb before feeling the limb, much of the objective information will be lost.

Feel

Palpation of the limb needs to be firm enough to elicit tenderness, but gentle enough not to cause the child undue pain and distress. This is a skill that the health care practitioner needs to practise before examining the child. Again, palpation of the limb needs to be in a logical and systematic way.

Limb palpation

(Advanced skill)

The joint above (proximal to the injury) is initially palpated to ensure that there is no bony tenderness.

- Locate all of the bony landmarks of this joint.
- Slowly and systemically move towards the injury, palpating bony prominences.
- Always observe the reaction of the child.

Once the child complains of tenderness the practitioner should stop and then palpate the injury distal to the injury, continuing to observe the child and stopping when the child complains of pain.

Only by completing a systematic examination will the practitioner ensure that no associated injuries are missed. Determine:

- area of maximum bony tenderness;
- area of ligamentous tenderness;
- any associated crepitus (rubbing of bone resembling a crackling noise);
- associated swelling;

- haematomas;
- associated lacerations;
- heat around the joint.

Due to the age of the child sometimes it will be difficult to determine the area of maximal tenderness, and on occasions the practitioner may have to request a radiograph of the whole limb if unable to determine the exact area of maximal bony tenderness.

Warmth of joint/limb
(Basic skill)
Always:

- palpate for warmth of the joint with the palm or back of your hand;
- compare with the other limb.

Any obvious joint heat can indicate that an inflammatory process is occurring. Arthritis is a common paediatric complaint and manifests by the presence of classical signs of:

- redness
- heat
- pain
- swelling
- loss of function.

Move
(Advanced skill)
The 'look' and 'feel' sections of the examination will help the health care practitioner to isolate the injured area. It is movement that give clues to the exact structure involved (Wardrope & English 1998). There are various ranges of movement:

- active (child is able to do by him-/herself)
- passive (health care practitioner moves the joint within the normal range of movement)
- resistance
- stress.

When examining children, always perform active movements before passive movements. If you do it the other way round then you may hurt the child and that is then the end of your examination (Gill & O'Brien 1998). In small children it is very easy to watch the child moving (or not moving!) the affected limb. Get the child to move the limb by offering a toy to the child for him or her to take, or watch the child playing or moving around the examination room. Then passively move the limb within the limits of the child's pain threshold.

In testing resisted movement, the joints do not move but the child presses against the practitioner's hand to test specific muscle groups. Pain on such movement indicates that the musculotendon is the site of the problem (Wardrope & English 1998). However, resisted movements of the joint can only be performed on children that are able to understand what is required.

- With infants, it may be impossible to test resistance completely.
- In toddlers, make the movement into a game to try to encourage the child to cooperate in the examination.
- Children over the age of 5 years should be able to complete resisted movements; however, this will require careful instructions to the child.

Stress testing abnormal movement indicates that the normal factors maintaining stability have been significantly damaged. However, it must be remembered that muscle power is one of the major factors influencing the stability of the joint. In the injured child, reflex muscle spasm may prevent the demonstration of ligamentous instability. If instability is to be demonstrated, then the child must be as relaxed as possible (Wardrope & English 1998). This can be very difficult to achieve in the child that is in pain and scared. Therefore, it can be impossible to fully assess the extent of ligamentous damage.

When examining the movement of the injured limb it needs to be done discretely. If the limb or joint is grossly deformed and the health care practitioner suspects that there is an underlying fracture then DO NOT move the limb just to ascertain the presence of crepitus and confirm the presence of a fracture; this is not good practice.

Table 12.3 Normal range of movements of the joints.

Upper limbs	Lower limbs
Shoulder	*Hip*
Abduction 0–180°	Flexion 110–120°
Forward flexion 0–180°	Extension 30°
Internal rotation 0–90°	Abduction 50°
External rotation 0–70°	Adduction 30°
Elbow	Internal rotation 45°
Flexion 0–150°	External rotation 45°
Supination 0–90°	*Knee*
Pronation 0–80°	Flexion 135°
Wrist	Hyperextension 10°
Flexion 75°	*Ankle*
Dorsiflexion 70°	Flexion 48°
Radial deviation 20°	Extension 18°
Ulnar deviation 30°	*Subtalar*
Pronation 70°	Inversion 5°
Supination 85°	Eversion 5°
Fingers	*Midtarsal*
Metacarpophalangeal (MCP) joint	Inversion 33°
Flexion 90°	Eversion 18°
Extension 45°	
Proximal interphalangeal (IP) joint	
Flexion 100°	
Distal IP joint	
Flexion 80°	
Thumb	
IP joint 0–80°	
First MCP joint 0–50°	

Testing joint movements requires knowledge of the normal range of movement of the joints. Table 12.3 shows this.

NEUROVASCULAR ASSESSMENT

Neurovascular assessment consists of examination of the nervous system (see Chapter 6) and vascular system (see Chapter 4) distal to the injury. To assess the vascular system (basic skill):

- Palpate the pulses distally to the injury, e.g. in supracondylar fractures both the radial and ulnar pulses must be palpated to ensure adequate circulation and perfusion of the distal limb.
- Colour and warmth of the limb must be assessed and compared with the uninjured limb. If there are no pulses present and the limb is pale and cool to touch it could indicate vascular compromise. This can occur if the joint is dislocated; if the distal limb has vascular compromise then the joint needs to be relocated as quickly as possible. If the situation dictates then the joint will be reduced prior to obtaining radiographs. However, it must be remembered that joint dislocation is rare in children and, therefore, the likelihood of vascular compromise is also rare.

Assessment of the neurological status of the limbs (advanced skill) (see Chapter 7) needs an understanding of normal neurology. The peripheral nerves of the upper limbs consist of the radial nerve, median nerve and ulnar nerve:

- The radial nerve supplies the triceps and brachioradialis and the extensor muscles of the hand. To test the radial nerve ask the child to flex the elbow, pronate the elbow and then extend the wrist. The radial nerve innervates the area surrounding the anatomical snuff box.
- The median nerve contains the motor supply to all the muscles on the front of the forearm. Therefore, to assess the motor supply of the median nerve ask the child to oppose the thumb to the little finger. The sensory component of the median nerve covers the palmar aspect of the thumb, index, middle and half of the ring finger.
- The ulnar nerve enters the forearm from the posterior to the medial epicondyle of the humerus. It innervates the muscles of the forearm, the hypothenar muscles, the seven interosseous muscles and the muscles to the ring and little finger. The ulnar nerve is a common nerve to be damaged if the child has an elbow injury, such as a supracondylar fracture. Therefore the sensory component of the ulnar nerve covers the dorsum and palmar aspects of the little and half ring finger.

Neurovascular examination depends upon the child's age. If the child is old enough, the practitioner will be able to accurately assess the neurovascular status of the injured limb. However, if the child is younger and unable to articulate or comply with the examination then it will be more difficult to assess the neurovascular status.

- Normal skin should be slightly moist (basic skill). Nerve dysfunction can cause a loss of sympathetic innervation in the area of distribution, and the skin becomes dry (American Society for Surgery of the Hand 1990). This is of clinical help in assessing nerve dysfunction, especially in children when the assessment can be difficult. In younger children the use of the 'immersion test' may be of benefit. An innervated hand or foot will wrinkle if submerged in water for 5–10 minutes. Failure of the skin to wrinkle may be suggestive of nerve dysfunction (American Society for Surgery of the Hand 1990).
- In older children it may be possible to complete the two-point discrimination test (see Chapter 6 for technique) (advanced skill). An abnormal distance is greater than 6 mm (American Society for Surgery of the Hand 1990). This could indicate nerve dysfunction.

When examining the lower limb, if the child is weight bearing the gait must be observed. This will give good information regarding the tone and muscle strength of the lower limbs.

The peripheral nerves of the lower limb include the lateral cutaneous nerve of the thigh, femoral nerve, sciatic nerve and the common perineal nerve (advanced skill):

- The lateral cutaneous nerve of the thigh should be assessed for sensory loss on the lateral aspect of the thigh.
- The femoral nerve is assessed by hip flexion and extension of the knee.
- The sciatic nerve supplies all of the muscles below the knee and some of the hamstrings. The loss of the sciatic nerve can cause foot drop and weakness in knee flexion.
- The common perineal nerve terminates from the sciatic nerve. It supplies the anterior and lateral compartments of the

muscles of the leg. Therefore the perineal nerve can be tested by looking for weakness in dorsiflexion and eversion of the foot (Talley & O'Connor 2001). Again, two-point discrimination can be used for older children and the immersion test can be used with younger children.

Common bedside monitoring
(Basic skill)

Following the admission of a child with a musculoskeletal injury, it is common to use the acronym 'CWSP' to assess the neurovascular system distal to the injury/plaster:

- C (colour): note the colour (pink, pale, cyanosed).
- W (warmth): note the temperature (hot, warm, cool).
- S (sensation): can the child feel an induced sensation, e.g. a sharp object pushed against the skin?
- P (pulses): note the volume of the pulse (0 nil, 1 weak, 2 normal, 3 bounding).

Your local assessment tool may also ask you to assess the capillary refill time (CRT) and oedema (see Chapter 4), motor activity (see Chapter 6) and pain (see Chapter 14).

Check that the assessment is undertaken frequently at first (e.g. hourly), decreasing as clinically indicated (e.g. 4–6 hourly), according to local policy.

Health care practitioners must also assess for compartment syndrome (compromised blood supply increasing the risk of ischaemia and necrosis). Compartment syndrome (using the 5 P's) is characterised by:

- Pain: pain that is increasing despite any relieving factors.
- Pallor: the skin is becoming pale.
- Paraesthesia: tingling or 'pins and needles' sensation.
- Paralysis: numbness/loss of feeling.
- Pulselessness: pulses have become weak and then are lost.

SUMMARY

In assessing a child with a musculoskeletal problem the health care practitioner may need to adapt some of the examination techniques to the age and co-operation of the child. It is essential that the examiner has clear history, including mechanism of injury, if applicable. Be acutely aware of non-accidental injury of children presenting with musculoskeletal problems.

When examining the child a logical and systematic assessment using *look, feel, move* should be completed. This will ensure that the entire limb is examined and that no other injuries or conditions are missed. Lastly, the neurovascular status of the limb should be assessed. Again the health care practitioner may need to adapt the examination according to the child's age.

REFERENCES

American Society for Surgery of the Hand (1990) *The Hand Examination and Diagnosis*, 3rd edn. Churchill Livingstone, London.

Giardino, A. (2006) *Child Abuse and Neglect: Physical Abuse*. www.emedicine.com/ped/topic2648.htm.

Gill, D. & O'Brien, N. (1998) *Paediatric Clinical Examination*, 3rd edn. Churchill Livingstone, London.

Glasgow, J. & Graham, H. (1997) *Management of Injuries in Children*. British Medical Journal Books, London.

Guly, H. (1996) *History Taking, Examination, and Record Keeping in Emergency Medicine*. Oxford University Press, Oxford.

Kay, L., Baggott, G., Coady, D. & Foster, J. (2003) Musculoskeletal examination for children and adolescents: do standard textbooks contain enough information? *Rheumatology*, **42**, 1423–1425.

Morton, R. & Phillips, B. (1992) *Accidents and Emergencies in Children*. Oxford University Press, Oxford.

Talley, N. & O'Connor, S. (2001) *Clinical Examination: A Systematic Guide to Physical Diagnosis*, 4th edn. Blackwell Publishing, Oxford.

Thornton, A. & Gyll, C. (1999) *Children's Fracture*. W.B Saunders, London.

Wardrope, J. & English, B. (1998) *Musculo-skeletal Problem in Emergency Medicine*. Oxford University Press, Oxford.

13 | Temperature Monitoring

INTRODUCTION

Temperature monitoring aims to assess the body's core (brain, visceral organs and tissues in the trunk) temperature. Under normal circumstances the patient's core temperature remains fairly constant, despite environmental changes, with the exception of the infant who has an immature thermoregulatory mechanism. However, the physiological mechanisms the body uses to maintain temperature may be detrimental to the sick infant and young child (Moore 2003). Further, young children, infants and acutely ill patients are unable to communicate or alter their environment in response to feeling cold or warm. Monitoring the temperature will therefore assist the health care practitioner in determining the appropriate warming and cooling/temperature-reduction technique required.

LEARNING OBJECTIVES

By the end of this chapter the reader will be able to:

❏ Understand the concepts of thermoregulation, cold and warm stress and neutral thermal environments.
❏ Use physical assessment techniques in identifying characteristics of hypothermia and hyperthermia.
❏ Review the differing techniques of assessing the core body temperature.
❏ Understand the mechanism, rationale and use of warming and cooling/temperature-reduction techniques.

PHYSICAL EXAMINATION

Temperature assessment and monitoring includes the physical examination of many systems, including:

• posture: curled up/extended;
• skin: cutaneous vasoconstriction/dilation;

- body hair: piloerection at lower temperatures;
- muscular activity: shivering, moving;
- respiratory system (see Chapter 2);
- cardiovascular system (see Chapter 4);
- neurological system: cranial nerves and coma scoring (see Chapters 7 and 11);
- renal system (see Chapter 10).

Heat is produced by the body as a by-product of cell metabolism. The hypothalamus controls thermoregulation (Kapit *et al*. 2000). Normothermia is considered to be 36.5–37.5°C. This normal range varies between individuals and is influenced by the time of day (Kapit *et al*. 2000), level of activity, drug therapy and gender. The normal range can also vary between different measurement tools; check manufacturer's guidelines. To compare temperature readings, these should be taken in the same place with the same tool each time and documented.

Due to the larger body surface area to body weight ratio, larger head to body ratio, lower nutritional stores and immature organ function, heat is lost from the body in infants and children more easily. Table 13.1 shows the mechanisms of heat loss and gain (Thomas 1994; WHO 1997).

When the patient's temperature begins to increase or decrease, as recognised by skin receptors (Kapit *et al*. 2000), look for changes in behaviour and physiology (basic skill), as follows.

Behaviour

- Altered posture: the child will change position to increase or decrease the amount of heat lost by convection and radiation.
  - Look for a curled up (to conserve heat) or extended (to lose heat) posture.
- Activity: this will increase or decrease muscle tone to increase or decrease heat production.
  - Look for lethargy (to decrease muscle tone) or increased activity (e.g. stamping feet, rubbing body, to increase muscle tone).
- Skin blood flow: this decreases or increases the amount of heat lost by convection and radiation.

Table 13.1 Mechanisms of heat loss and gain.

Mechanism	Heat is lost from	Heat is gained from
Convection	Skin to surrounding air, e.g. cool room and corridors, drafts from air vents, windows, doors, fans, air conditioners Cold oxygen flow	Surrounding air to skin, e.g. hot day, room heater, heated incubator, isolette
Radiation	Skin to nearest surface that faces the skin, independent of surrounding air temperature, e.g. cold incubator walls Being near windows, cold external walls, single-walled incubators	Nearby surface that faces the skin, independent of surrounding air temperature, e.g. sun, heat lamps
Conduction	Skin to surface in direct contact, e.g. cold mattress, blanket, weighing scales, table, X-ray plate, clothing	A surface in direct contact with the skin, e.g. warm mattress, heating pads, hot water bottles, chemical bags, skin-to-skin contact including 'kangaroo care'
Evaporation	As water evaporates from skin and lungs By insensible water loss (at lower temperatures) By sweating (at higher temperatures) e.g. a wet baby after delivery or with washing, application of lotions, solutions, wet packs or soaks	Warm moist gases, e.g. humidified environment including incubator, and humidified piped gases including ventilation circuits

- o Look for cutaneous vasoconstriction (conserves heat) or dilation (loses heat).

Physiology

- Sweating: sweat glands increase fluid loss and subsequent evaporative heat loss; this is not well developed in the neonate.
  - o Look for patches of damp on the skin, electrolyte imbalance and dehydration (see Chapter 10).

- Shivering: this increases heat production by involuntary contraction of muscles; it is not well developed in the neonate.
  - Look for increased heart rate, acidosis and hypoxia in the sick child or infant.
- Sympathetic stimulation: this
  - increases cellular metabolism and heat production in the child.
  - Look for increased heart rate, acidosis and respiratory distress in the sick child or infant.
  - metabolises brown adipose tissue for heat production in the neonate. This is known as non-shivering thermogenesis. Supplies of brown fat and glycogen are limited, and thus temperature falls.
    - Look for respiratory distress, hypoxia, acidosis and hypoglycaemia in the sick neonate.

HYPERTHERMIA

A high temperature is due to:

- Fever: the temperature set-point in the hypothalamus is raised (and becomes the new 'normal') in response to an infection. Infants and children respond with behavioural and physiological changes as if they are cold, i.e. they increase heat production and therefore their temperature.
  - Look for (basic skill): high temperature (neonates may have hypothermia in response to infection), cool hands and feet, pale skin, lethargy, looking unwell.
  - Treat by restoring the set-point, e.g. give Brufen.
- Overheating: as a response to a change in the environmental temperature. The infant and child respond with behavioural and physiological responses in order to increase heat loss and lower body temperature.
  - Look for (basic skill): high temperature, warm hands and feet, pink skin, extended posture, does not necessarily look unwell.
  - Treat by reducing the environmental temperature.
- Drug fever:
  - some drugs raise the temperature, e.g. phenytoin, histamine blockers, procainamide, antibiotics (Pate 2001);

- may raise basal metabolic rate (BMR), increase skeletal muscle activity and lower cutaneous blood flow;
- may take up to 5 days to resolve.

HYPOTHERMIA

Infants or children who do not respond normally to stimulation without an adequate explanation should be assessed for hypothermia (Pate 2001). There are various levels of hypothermia. Table 13.2 outlines what to assess for (basic skill).

Drug pharmacodynamics and pharmacokinetics

Some drugs that your patient may be on can have an effect on thermal regulation:

- Phenothiazines (anti-psychotic drugs, e.g. chlorpromazine) and barbiturates have a direct effect on the anterior hypothalamus, thereby decreasing its ability to respond to cold.
- Neuroblocking agents and phenothiazines decrease the ability to shiver.
- Vasodilators inhibit peripheral vasoconstriction and excess heat can be lost (Brink 1990).

If your patient is hypothermic, it may have an impact on how certain drugs work:

- Due to the slow metabolic rate and biochemical reactions you will be less able to evaluate drug levels and their effects.
- Due to decreased cardiac output, dehydration, slowed hepatic metabolism, impaired glomerular filtration rate, abnormal renal tubular filtration and reabsorption, drug clearance may be reduced. Moreover, hypothermia:
  - elevates the toxic dose of digoxin;
  - decreases inotrope dose;
  - at mildly low levels may enhance catecholamine effects, but at moderate to severe levels decreases catecholamine effects;
  - causes electrolyte-induced arrhythmias;
  - heightens sensitivity to anaesthetics and barbiturates (Brink 1990).

Table 13.2 Levels of hypothermia and what to assess for.

Level/temperature	Consequences/assess for
Mild hypothermia 32–36°C	Cool skin and pallor
	Shivering at 30–35°C; becomes uncontrolled
	Mental confusion, drowsiness, restlessness, disorientation
	Tachycardia; may start to become bradycardic
	Tachypnoea; may start to become bradypnoeic
	Resuscitation may not be effective; resuscitation should continue until temperature is at least above 32°C
	The hypothalamus is not functioning well (Pate 2001)
Moderate hypothermia 28–32°C	Below 30°C the hypothalamus is not working and there is rapid temperature loss and death ensues (Pate 2001)
	Shivering stops
	Confusion/slowness, vague and slurred speech and changes in neurological state due to a decrease in cerebral blood flow (Pate 2001)
	Significant decrease in metabolic rate
	Hypoventilation with some apnoea
	Hypoxia and acidosis
	Cold diuresis: cannot concentrate urine, and dehydration ensues (Brink 1990)
	Further cardiac arrhythmias, e.g. atrial fibrillation and ventricular arrhythmias
Deep hypothermia 17–27.7°C	Heart block (second degree progressing to complete heart block)
	Coma
	Apnoea
	Fixed dilated pupils
Profound hypothermia 4–16.5°C	Hypothermia may be induced for cardiac surgery, but cardiopulmonary support systems are put in place, e.g. cardiopulmonary bypass

TEMPERATURE-MONITORING TOOLS

Selection of your tool will depend upon availability, training, the seriousness of the illness of the infant and child and how much monitoring is required. Table 13.3 shows the different tools available and the assessment required for each.

Table 13.3 Temperature monitoring tools and assessment required for each.

Tool	Comments	Check for
Pulmonary artery (PA) Used when a PA catheter is in situ (see Chapter 3) (advanced skill)	Considered to be the gold standard PA is closest to the carotid arteries that supply the hypothalamus, so is closely correlated to core temperature Invasive	All the complications of a PA catheter (see Chapter 5)
Bladder Used in patients following major surgery, e.g. cardiac surgery (advanced skill)	Closely correlates with PA (Lefrant et al. 2003) Built into the indwelling bladder catheter Invasive	All the complications of a urethral catheter
Oesophageal/nasopharyngeal Used in the operating theatre, e.g. during cardiac surgery (advanced skill)	Oesophageal correlates well with PA and bladder temperatures Invasive	All the complications of an intragastric tube (see Chapter 9)
Rectal Used in critically ill children and historically in infants (advanced skill)	Slow response to changes in temperature due to limited blood supply and thermoreceptors in rectum and greater distance from rectum to hypothalamus Concerns with accuracy at high and low temperatures (Morgan et al. 2001) Faeces can impact on results Invasive	Patient discomfort Rectal perforations (Wolfson 1996) Vagal stimulation and bradycardia (Bailey & Rose 2000) Correct depth of placement (3 cm) Adequate dwell time (3–5 minutes)

Tympanic
Most commonly used
(basic skill)

Close correlation with core temperature with a stable temperature or changing temperature (Nimah *et al.* 2006); more accurate than rectal, forehead or axilla monitoring

The common carotid artery provides blood supply to the tympanic membrane as well as hypothalamus. As there is little metabolic tympanic activity, temperature reflects blood supply

Child co-operation, wax and infection have been shown not to impact on results (Chamberlain *et al.* 1991; Terndrup & Wong 1991)

Protected from impact of ambient temperature

Preferred choice of children compared with axillary or digital thermometry (Pickersgill 1997)

Non-invasive

Correct technique following manufacturer's recommendations must be employed:

- gently pulling ear back in infants and 'up and back' in children to expose tympanic membrane to probe
- knowing the recommendations for certain groups to repeat the measures, e.g. infants
- if child has been lying on the ear used for temperature taking, turn patient and wait a few minutes prior to taking temperature

Axilla and forehead
Commonly used at home
(basic skill)

Less accurate; affected by environmental temperature and changes in skin perfusion (Cusson *et al.* 1997)

Axilla and temporal artery measurements provide similar accuracy (Hebbar *et al.* 2005)

Under-reads core temperature and inconsistent readings possible (Nimah *et al.* 2006)

Non-invasive

Accurate application of technique: good skin contact with thermometer at apex of axilla or across forehead

Patient discomfort

Continued

303

Table 13.3 *Continued.*

Tool	Comments	Check for
Oral Historically commonly used in acute and non-acute settings (basic skill)	Poor accuracy and affected by: • hyperventilation • position of probe • recent cool or warm drinks • a child who cannot close mouth properly (Terndrup *et al.* 1989) • oral temperature normally 0.5°C lower than core temperature Non-invasive	Accurate application of technique: placed in sublingual pocket under tongue on either side of frenulum Patient discomfort
Peripheral Reflects regional temperature rather than core temperature and therefore subject to vasomotor and environmental impact Used in acute care (advanced skill)	Placed on abdomen or chest for servo-control warming in the incubator or radiant heater Placed on feet/toes to measure difference between core temperature and regional temperature; indicative of cardiac output and perfusion	Attached to abdomen or back, avoiding bony prominences (Leick-Rude & Bloom 1998) Infant is not lying on probe (Blackburn *et al.* 2001a,b) Change probe site and cover when becoming loose (Blackburn *et al.* 2001a,b) Assess old site for epidermal damage Well secured (as recommended by manufacturer) May need securing to the patient proximally to reduce tension on probe Pressure areas

Table 13.4 Warming/cooling methods and their assessment.

Method	Comments	Check for
Appropriate clothing (basic skill)	Hats and bonnets for babies as 75% of heat loss is through the head	Appropriateness of clothing
Foil blankets Also known as • emergency blanket • space blanket • silver swaddler • reflective foil (advanced skill)	Used in an emergency, e.g. road traffic accident, drowning or at birth Prevents further heat loss but does not warm patient Patient can sweat (impermeable material), increasing heat loss Effectiveness not known	Cannot observe patient so undertake physical examination as required Skin allergies Environment, as blanket is flammable
Water mattress/heated mattress – infant (advanced skill)	Used in the stable baby May be used for the infant who previously was nursed in an incubator and is now 'normalising' as much as possible Easy access for parents and carers Provides conductive heat	The temperature that is actually needed Pressure areas Core temperature monitoring It is left on between use as it takes a long time to heat up
Forced air warmers Also known as • warming blanket (basic skill)	Used in acute care settings Different shapes and sizes available Draws room air through a filter and warms (or cools) the air to a specified temperature and creates a warm environment by conduction and convection Note that this technique can be used to provide a warm environment for the sick	Cannot observe patient so undertake physical examination as required Vital signs as blanket can work quickly Core temperature monitoring – often a rectal probe, but does not have to be Perfusion of patient as there may be thermal injury to ischaemic limbs Blanket is anchored if necessary

Continued

Table 13.4 Continued.

Method	Comments	Check for
	child but it cannot (and should not be used to) override pathophysiological states, e.g. the shocked patient who is peripherally cold	
Heating pads Also known as • transwarmer (advanced skill)	Used in <10-kg infants (above this, ratio of body surface area to body mass is insufficient to achieve reasonable benefit) Often used for transport Heat is produced by a chemical reaction and warms patient by conduction, convection and radiation	Core temperature monitoring as temperature of pad cannot be regulated Temperature of blanket as it will cool when the heat has dissipated Activate just before use for maximum time (usually lasts several hours) Remove prior to MRI scanning (metal button)
Incubators (advanced skill)	Used for neonates who are born prematurely or who have undergone surgery or as a staged return to normal following a critical care event The warm air provides convective heat Adding heat shields may prevent convective or evaporative losses Uses servo control by attaching a probe to abdomen or chest; incubator will provide heat to make the air the same temperature as the set temperature	If infant is clothed/partially clothed full observation is difficult so undertake physical examination as required Core temperature monitoring Phototherapy management if used Humidification system if used – reduces evaporative heat losses in premature infants (Rutter 1995) Signs of infection Oxygenation monitoring if used All access points closed and only opened when necessary for procedures Appropriate height for parents and carers

Also uses a manual control where a consistent temperature is set despite the infant's own temperature

Consider bonding strategies to overcome physical barrier

Ensure the top is not used for storage of equipment or tapped on as this is very noisy for the infant

Close observation of infant as he/she may not be able to be heard

It is not placed in direct sunlight as this will cause a 'greenhouse' effect

It is not placed in a cool, draughty room as this will have an impact on ability of incubator to warm baby

Incubator is pre-warmed prior to placing an infant in there

You may want to place your stethoscope head in the incubator to keep it warm

Pressure area from probe site

Radiant heaters

Also known as

• overhead heaters

(advanced skill)

Used in critically ill infants where easy and quick access is required

Provides heat by radiation but increased loss of heat by evaporation (Loughead et al. 1997)

Uses servo control by attaching a probe to the abdomen or chest; heater will provide heat to make the air the same temperature as the set temperature

Also uses a manual control where a consistent temperature is set despite infant's own temperature

Core temperature monitoring; often with a rectal probe but does not necessarily have to be

Eyes for damage

Skin for signs of flash burns

Fluid status for excess insensible water loss

Phototherapy management if used

Resuscitation facilities if available

Pressure areas from probe site

It is not placed in a cool and draughty place, increasing the risk of heat loss by convection and radiation. You may want to use clingfilm to cover corners and over top of infant

There is as little interference with heat source as possible as infant's temperature will quickly drop, e.g. chest X-rays, interventions and procedures

Continued

Table 13.4 *Continued.*

Method	Comments	Check for
		Parents can gain access to the baby
		That infant is not overly handled due to easy access
		Light source can be used for procedures but this is very bright and you may need to protect infant's eyes
		It is pre-warmed prior to placing baby in it
		Staff and parents are aware of the heat on their heads when standing for long periods under the heater
		Problems are attended to quickly as alarms can be noisy and startling to infant
		No oils or creams are used on the baby as this will increase risk of burning
		Heater is positioned in a quiet part of the room as there is no protection from external noise for infant
Heating/cooling mattress – children (advanced skill)	Used less often nowadays in critical care as there is no evidence for hypothermic management in head-injured patients (Adelson *et al.* 2003) Mattress has water which is warmed or cooled to a pre-set degree	Vital signs as it can work quickly Core temperature monitoring; often a rectal probe but does not necessarily have to be Place layers of linen between patient and mattress to prevent cold and hot burns Check frequently for pressure areas The non-chemically restrained patient may shiver in response to cooling thereby negating the effect

Efforts are made to assist the infant, young child and acutely ill patient by maintaining an appropriate environment. A neutral thermal environment is one where core temperature is maintained without the need for behavioural or physiological responses, thereby reducing the negative impact of these responses (Thomas 1994). Table 13.4 shows different warming and cooling devices/methods and how to assess these.

SUMMARY
Temperature assessment and management is important in infants and children, especially those who are sick. Different tools have different accuracy in monitoring and therefore have implications for management. The infant and in particular the neonate is at high risk of severe morbity with hypothermia.

REFERENCES
Adelson, P.D., Bratton, S.L., Carney, N.A., *et al.* (2003) Guidelines for the acute medical management of severe traumatic brain injury in infants, children and adolescents. *Pediatric Critical Care Medicine*, **4** (3) (Suppl.).

Bailey, J. & Rose, P. (2000) Temperature measurement in the preterm infant: a literature review. *Journal of Neonatal Nursing*, **6** (1), 28–32.

Blackburn, S., DePaul, D., Loan, L.A., *et al.* (2001a) Neonatal thermal care, part II: microbial growth under temperature probe covers. *Neonatal Network*, **20** (3), 19–22.

Blackburn, S., DePaul, D., Loan, L.A., *et al.* (2001b) Neonatal thermal care, part III: the effect of infant position and temperature probe placement. *Neonatal Network*, **20** (3), 25–30.

Brink, L.W. (1990) Abnormalities in temperature regulation. In: Levin, D.L. & Morriss, F.C. (eds) *Essentials of Pediatric Intensive Care*. Quality Medical Publishing, St. Louis.

Chamberlain, J.M., Grandner, J. & Rubinoff, J.L. (1991) Comparison of a tympanic thermometer to rectal and oral thermometers in a pediatric emergency department. *Clinical Pediatrics*, **30**, 24–29.

Cusson, R.M., Madonia, J.A. & Taekman, J.B. (1997) The effect of environment on body site temperatures in full-term neonates. *Nursing Research*, **46**, 202–207.

Hebbar, K., Fortenberry, J.D., Rogers, K., Merritt, R. & Easley, K. (2005) Comparison of temporal artery thermometer to standard temperature measurements in paediatric intensive care unit patients. *Pediatric Critical Care Medicine*, **6** (5), 557–561.

Kapit, N., Macey, R. & Meisami, E. (2000) *The Physiology Coloring Book*. Addison Wesley Longman, San Francisco.

Lefrant, J.Y., Muller, L., Coussaye, J.E., *et al.* (2003) Temperature measurement in intensive care patients: comparison of urinary bladder, esophageal, rectal, axillary and inguinal methods versus pulmonary artery core method. *Intensive Care Medicine*, **29** (3), 414–418.

Leick-Rude, M.K. & Bloom, L.F. (1998) A comparison of temperature-taking methods in neonates. *Neonatal Network*, **17** (5), 21–37.

Loughead, M.K., Loughead, J.L. & Reinhart, M.J. (1997) Incidence and physiological characteristics of hypothermia in the very low birth weight infant. *Paediatric Nursing*, **23** (1), 11–15.

Moore, J. (2003) From birth to neonatal unit: a cold journey? *Journal of Neonatal Nursing*, Step-by-Step Guide.

Morgan, G., Mikhail, M. & Murray, M. (eds) (2001) *Clinical Anesthesiology*. McGraw Hill, New York.

Nimah, M.N., Bshesh, K., Callahan, J.D. & Jacobs, B.R. (2006) Infrared tympanic thermometry in comparison with other temperature measurement techniques in febrile children. *Pediatric Critical Care Medicine*, **7** (1), 48–55.

Pate, M.F.D. (2001) Thermal regulation. In: Curley, M.A.Q & Moloney-Harmon, P.A. (eds) *Critical Care Nursing of Infants and Children*, 2nd edn. W.B. Saunders, Philadelphia.

Pickersgill, J. (1997) Taking the pressure off. *Paediatric Nursing*, **9** (8), 25–27.

Rutter, N. (1995) *A Guide to Incubator Care*. Vickers Medical Ltd., Sidcup.

Terndrup, T.E. & Wong, A. (1991) Influence of otitis media on the correlation between rectal and auditory canal temperatures. *American Journal of Diseases in Childhood*, **145**, 75–78.

Terndrup, T.E., Allegra, J.R. & Kealy, J.A. (1989) A comparison of oral, rectal and tympanic membrane-derived temperature changes after ingestion of liquids and smoking. *American Journal of Emergency Medicine*, **7**, 150–154.

Thomas, K. (1994) Thermoregulation in neonates. *Neonatal Network*, **13** (2), 15–22.

Wolfson, J.S. (1996) Rectal perforation in infants by thermometer. *American Journal of Diseases in Childhood*, **111**, 197–200.

World Health Organisation (WHO) (1997) *Safe Motherhood: Thermal Protection of the Newborn: A Practical Guide*. World Health Organisation, Geneva.

Comfort and Hygiene

14

INTRODUCTION

Sick and critically ill children are cared for in an environment that is alien, interrupts their normal routine, interferes with normal growth and development and demands unpleasant interventions and procedures. The aim of this chapter is to outline assessment techniques to help maintain comfort and hygiene.

LEARNING OBJECTIVES

By the end of this chapter the reader will be able to:

❑ Explore the assessment of skin integrity.
❑ Appreciate adapted hygiene activities.
❑ Assess intravenous catheter sites.
❑ Administer appropriate therapy through sedation and pain scoring.
❑ Recognise the impact of the environment on the sick child.

SKIN INTEGRITY

Skin damage due to pressure occurs when soft tissue is squashed between a bony prominence and an external hard surface; capillary blood flow is decreased resulting in ischaemia and necrosis to the area. Check for increased risk of occurrence (basic skill).

• Intrinsic factors include oedema, hypothermia, dehydration, sepsis, some medications, e.g. inotropes, immobility, poor perfusion, anaemia, incontinence, pain and sedation, decreased weight for age and poor nutrition (Pickersgill 1997).

- Extrinsic factors include:
  - extended time in one place and/or on a hard surface (pressure);
  - the epidermis of the skin is pulled in opposite direction to the underlying tissues, e.g. sitting upright or sliding down the bed (shearing);
  - the skin is pulled against another surface, e.g. pulling child up the bed; often associated with abrasions and blisters (friction);
  - lying in moisture, e.g. secretions, urine, gastric fluid, drainage and stools can cause bacterial growth and skin breakdown (moisture) (Waterlow 1998).

Check for the most common causes of skin breakdown (basic skill).

- In infants: the use of adhesives, nappy rash, friction, heat burns and infection in that order, and usually seen on arms and legs, trunk (back and front) and then face in that order (Lund *et al.* 2001b). The higher the number of devices attached to the infant, the higher the incidence of skin breakdown (Lund *et al.* 2001b).
- Occiput, ears and heels are common pressure sites in children (Curley *et al.* 2003a).

Risk assessment should be undertaken as soon as possible after admission. Some units have protocols on undertaking this and how often it should occur (Pickersgill 1997; Waterlow 1998; Curley *et al.* 2003b; Suddaby *et al.* 2005). Using a scale can give guidelines on which preventative strategies can be put in place, depending on the level of risk.

(*Note your clinical unit's guidelines here*:)

Check that (basic skill):

- Pressure is removed or reduced where possible; may need to use a pressure reducing/relieving mattress (RCN 2003b) or cushion (not always readily available for those under 20 kg).
- The child's skin is not left under pressure for any length of time; move or turn patient regularly (more regularly if the area becomes red; 2–3 hourly for high-risk patients).

- Staff have been trained in patient movement and transfer methods and that these are used appropriately.
- Transparent dressings are used to prevent shearing or friction forces.
- The child's skin is kept dry to prevent moisture accumulation.
- Risk areas are identified, e.g.
  - mechanical devices and probes attached to skin;
  - strapping attached to skin;
  - plaster/splints;
  - tubes lying against or through the skin, e.g. indwelling catheters, endotracheal tubes, masks, nasogastric tubes;
  - support strategies, e.g. roll under the neck or heels supported on devices;
  - forceps delivery (Waterlow 1997).

When tissue injury is identified, it can be classified into stages of breakdown (NICE 2005) (basic skill) so that appropriate treatment can be undertaken. Stages usually include:

1. reddened area with intact skin;
2. partial thickness skin loss, which may include blisters;
3. full thickness skin loss, also involving subcutaneous tissue;
4. deep tissue, which may include fascia.

Some units have protocols on undertaking this and how often it should occur (Bergstrom *et al.* 1994).

(*Note your clinical unit's guidelines here:*)

Assess for (basic skill):

- Redness or discoloration: increase movement or turning frequency or introduce pressure-relieving mattress.
- Skin breakdown: treat as a wound (see 'Wound Assessment' below).

SKIN HYGIENE
(Basic skill)
The sick child and infant require skin care that maintains normal skin function, including acting as a barrier (Fairley & Rasmussen 1983). Check:

- Bathing
  - Bathing should be undertaken two to three times per week, increasing to normal home pattern as the child recovers and moves about more.
  - Bathe at the time of soiling and nappy changes.
  - Bathe to remove blood and other body fluids.
  - Use a pH neutral soap substance (often liquid rather than bar to reduce risk of bar bacterial contamination) so that the skin pH is not altered too much (normally 6.34 at birth falling to 4.95 in first few days) (Lund *et al.* 1999).
  - Use a soap that has minimum perfume and dyes to try to prevent development of allergies.
  - Use the minimum soap quantity as all soaps are mildly irritating and dehydrating to the skin.
  - Emollients can be used to prevent skin breakdown by improving the barrier function of the infant's skin.
  - Chlorhexidine, iodine or other skin disinfectants are used only when specifically indicated, as chemicals are absorbed into the body through the skin; toxicity and skin damage (e.g. blister) can also occur (Lund *et al.* 2001a).
  - Physiological monitoring and clinical assessment for physiological instability are undertaken throughout the procedure, which is stopped if deterioration is noted (often by bradycardia and oxygen desaturation).
  - Bathing should not be prolonged so that the infant/child is at risk from hypothermia.
  - Excessive vernix on the newborn can be washed but does not have to be completely removed for hygiene reasons (it may actually have a protective function) (Lund *et al.* 1999).
  - Immersion bathing is probably better than sponging if at all possible as it is more soothing for the infant/child and will remove any creams, cells and adhesives as well as being more hydrating (Lund *et al.* 1999).
  - Skin should be gently dried and not rubbed harshly (as this removes epithelial cells and increases risk of skin breakdown).

- o The child/infant who is sweaty may need gentle sponging more often (eccrine glands open directly onto skin and are widely distributed).
- o Body odour in young people is a sensitive issue for them and more frequent washing, particularly in these areas, may be warranted. (Apocrine glands in the axilla and genital area open into hair follicles and are stimulated by emotional and physical stress; the bacterial decomposition of this sweat is responsible for the body odour (Bickley 2003).)
- The wash bowl is cleansed with disinfectant/alcohol and dried well in between use and placed where it cannot be contaminated (Skewes 1996).
- Using emollients can help counteract dry skin (take care not to use products associated with allergies), but use of emollients or moisturisers can be counterproductive when the infant is nursed in a warming device (see Chapter 13).
- Adhesive removal:
  - o Try to use barriers initially rather than tape directly onto the skin.
  - o Let adhesive consumables, e.g. ECG electrodes, fall off or wash off by themselves: replace only as necessary rather than routinely.
  - o Solvents can cause toxicity (Lund *et al*. 1999).

MOUTH CARE

Sick children will have decreased/ineffective saliva production so there is a greater risk of infection locally and systemically (bacteria transgress the highly vascularised gums). Check for causes:

- reduced mastication from not eating;
- decreased fluid intake;
- some drug administration;
- drying effects of mouth breathing;
- oxygen therapy;
- being nursed with their mouths open;
- an endotracheal tube in situ.

An endotracheal tube (ETT) or other tubes may cause pressure areas especially if the tube rests on the gingiva rather than the teeth. Micro-organisms from the mouth can migrate down these tubes, causing chest infections (Rubinstein *et al*. 1992) and possibly gastrointestinal infections (McNeil 2000).

Plaque that is not removed will lead to gingivitis. Mouth care is an all-encompassing term to ensure healthy buccal cavity tissue.

Assess (basic skill):

- Teeth and gum line: that they are clean with no plaque or debris.
- Gingiva: for pinkness and no inflammation or oedema (note oedema can be normal with childhood teething).
- Tongue: for a moist and pink surface with no coating.
- Mucous membranes: for moisture and pink surface and no dryness or ulceration.
- Saliva: for watery secretions and no thick tenacious or absent secretions.
- Lips: for softness and moistness with no dryness, cracking or bleeding (Gibson & Nelson 2000).
- Halitosis.

Check (basic skill):

- that a torch and gloved finger or tongue depressor is used to carefully examine all the surfaces of the buccal cavity, including under the tongue;
- an appropriate soft but small (ease of use) headed toothbrush is available for brushing of teeth (except for children with extensive ulceration or significantly abnormal clotting times (Ransier *et al*. 1995)) twice per day (best method of plaque removal);
- that toothpaste is available to make the brushing experience more pleasant and easier – rinse well as any alcohol in the paste has a drying effect;
- that foam swabs are:
  - used to help to remove loose debris and pooled secretions;
  - used to help moisten the mouth (up to every 2 hours) between brushing (Barnason *et al*. 1998);

- o dipped in water or normal saline as these are as effective as mouthwash (Feber 1995);
- o not used to primarily remove plaque;
- hydrogen peroxide appears to be harmful to the mucosa and is not recommended (Tombes & Galluci 1993) yet can successfully provide an antibacterial effect (Madeya 1996);
- that sodium bicarbonate is avoided as it alters the pH and can burn the mucosa (Kite & Pearson 1995);
- antibiotic solution may lead to resistance. However, when toothbrushes are absolutely impossible to use, foam swabs with chlorhexidene can be effective in removing plaque on a short-term basis (Ransier *et al.* 1995), but dilution must be accurate to prevent damage to the mucosa (Kite & Pearson 1995);
- artificial saliva can be used in the case of decreased saliva production (Madeya 1996).

EYE CARE

See 'Physical examination of the eyes' in Chapter 11. Children who have a decreased level of consciousness will have impaired (ineffective or reduced efficiency) corneal (blink) reflexes and be:

- unable to react to the potential threat of eye injury, increasing the risk of actual damage to the cornea;
- at risk of drying and infection of the cornea, with subsequent abrasions, ulceration and perforation.

Check for (basic skill):

- loss of corneal lustre
- dullness
- abnormal spots
- crusting
- inflammation.

Check that (basic skill):

- the eye is assessed every 2 hours when corneal or conjunctival dryness or infection has occurred and every 6 hours when there is no evidence of dryness;

- the eye is cleansed as required from inner to outer canthus, using sterile water or saline wiping very gently with cotton gauze (not cotton wool as wisps of cotton can scratch the cornea). Do not wipe the cornea itself.

The physiological effects of intubation and ventilation (fluid retention, increased venous and intraocular pressure) for the child who requires ventilatory assistance may predispose or exacerbate any ocular injury.

Check (advanced skill):

- that no respiratory secretions can accidentally lodge in the eyes;
- any securing techniques of tubes in and around the face, ensuring they are not too tight and compromising venous blood return from the head;
- for any objects near the eyes that can predispose to damage, e.g. strapping, gas flow from oxygen therapy or nasal CPAP (Gaili & Woodruff 2002);
- for oedema (orbital and lid) in and around the eyes that may decrease the ability to close the eye, with subsequent evaporation and dryness occurring.

An effective blink mechanism spreads tears evenly over the eye, providing moisture and cleansing, without which drying occurs. Check that evaporation is reduced in the unconscious child by (advanced skill):

- ensuring the eyes are kept closed:
  - using tape to secure the eye closed is a common practice but does not necessarily ensure complete eye closure (eye closure is normally accomplished by the orbicularis oculi muscle but this is affected by use of sedation and paralysis drugs). Also, skin can be damaged by the constant need to remove the tape for checking pupil response;
  - Gelliperm (polyacrylamide gel patch) is a transparent, soft, non-allergenic, water-based gel-like sheet that can be cut to size to cover the entire eye socket. Although it was developed for wound care in 1977 (Geistlich 1993), its current aims in eye care use include providing a barrier to infection

and a gentle pressure to maintain eyelid closure. It is easy to remove for eye inspection, but check that it is changed regularly when drying out; some local policies call for the rehydration of the patch (and therefore re-use (on same patient) with sterile water or saline;

(*Note your clinical unit's policy here:*)

o cling (polyethylene) film placed and secured over the eyes and orbits may create a moist environment to prevent corneal epithelial dryness and ulceration (Cortese *et al.* 1995);
o artificial tears ointment can be used to create a barrier between the eye; check that plenty of ointment is used and regularly topped up;
- providing moisture for the eyes (basic skill):
  o a commercial artificial tears solution can be soothing for dry eyes;
  o normal saline eye drops cause excessive tearing and eye irritation (Lloyd 1990) so should be used for irrigation only;
  o antibiotic eye drops should be used when an infection is evident and commenced only after taking an eye swab;
  o artificial tears ointment.

UMBILICAL CARE

The umbilical cord separates 5–15 days after birth and it is kept clean and dry with normal washing/bathing practice for normal healthy infants (Anderson 2004). Note that separation occurs by an inflammatory response and that white, sticky or slightly smelly mucus may be present during this process and for a few days until healing takes place.

Check (basic skill):

- the nappy is folded below the cord and left exposed to dry, or cover loosely with clean clothing (WHO 1998);
- the use of alcohol is discouraged as it can increase the period of time for the cord to separate (Dore *et al.* 1998);
- for inflammation (redness, swelling, pain), any offensive odour or discharge;

- the local policy for the use of antimicrobials, chlorhexidine or iodine within a nursery to reduce colonisation; however, these may delay cord separation.

INTRAVENOUS CATHETER ASSESSMENT

Intravenous (IV) catheters are frequently used for drug therapy, fluid administration, maintenance fluid, blood transfusions and nutrition in acutely sick children. The Royal College of Nursing (RCN 2003a) has published *Standards for Infusion Device Therapy*.

Check that (basic skill):

- the dressing is transparent;
- the dressing is not damp, loose or soiled;
- there is no blood or air in the catheter or tubing;
- the catheter and tubing are well secured;
- there is no leakage around the catheter due to:
  - patient movement;
  - inadequate stabilisation;
  - thrombosis;
  - a blood pressure cuff being used on the same limb.

Phlebitis

(Basic skill)

Phlebitis is an inflammation of the intima of the vein. A scale may be used to assess and manage phlebitis (see Fig. 14.1) (Jackson 1998).

Infiltration

(Basic skill)

Infiltration is the accidental administration of non-vesicant medications or solutions into the tissue rather than the vein. A scale may be used to assess and manage infiltration (Infusion Nurses Society 2006). The RCN *Standards for Infusion Device Therapy* (2003a) has an infiltration scale.

Extravasation

(Basic skill)

Extravasation is the leakage of a vesicant medication into sur-rounding tissue instead of the vein. Check for:

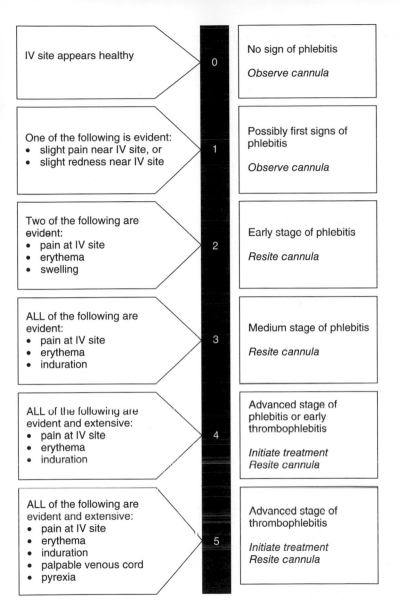

Fig. 14.1 Phlebitis assessment. (Reproduced courtesy of *Nursing Times*, Jackson, A. (1988) *Nursing Times*, **94** (4), 68–71.)

- blanching
- necrosis
- ulceration.

Extravasation is further assessed and managed as a wound often as part of an extravasation policy.

WOUND ASSESSMENT

There is a paucity of evidence in the literature outlining a paediatric wound scoring system.

For wounds that are healing by primary intention, e.g. surgical wounds, assess for (basic skill):

- no gaps in the wound;
- epithelialisation occurring at the site;
- no drainage;
- no evidence of infection;
- a palpable ridge along the wound.

(Doughty 2004)

For wounds healing by secondary intention, e.g. dehisced wounds or pressure areas, assess for (basic skill):

- M: measurement (size and depth);
- E: evidence of any exudate;
- A: appearance of the surrounding skin; any oedema, cellulitis or breakdown;
- S: suffering of any pain;
- U: any undermining of the wound edges, i.e. wound edges turn inwards so that they cannot align;
- R: redness or signs of infection;
- E: enlarging or getting smaller.

SEDATION SCORING

Sedative drugs depress the central nervous system, reducing mental activity and inducing sleep, and are used to promote comfort (reduce discomfort from physical and psychological causes), limit anxiety and agitation (from hypoxia or sensory imbalance) and promote safety (allow therapeutic procedures).

Children may require different levels of sedation. Check (basic skill):

- Conscious sedation:
  - protective reflexes and patent airways are maintained independently;
  - the child can respond to stimulation.
- Deep sedation:
  - airway patency requires support as it is partially or totally lost;
  - child not easily aroused.
- General anaesthesia:
  - protective reflexes are lost;
  - patent airway cannot be maintained;
  - no response to stimuli.

Appropriate sedation levels may be assessed by using a tool. Table 14.1 shows the Comfort Score (advanced skill). The use of blood pressure and pulse as variables has been challenged as they are non-specific signs of anxiety (Carnevale & Razack 2002).

Table 14.1 The Comfort Score.

Criteria	Score
Alertness	
Deeply asleep	1
Lightly asleep	2
Drowsy	3
Fully awake and alert	4
Hyperalert	5
Calmness/agitation	
Calm	1
Slightly anxious	2
Anxious	3
Very anxious	4
Panicky	5
Respiratory response	
No coughing/no spontaneous breaths	1
Spontaneous respiration with little or no response to ventilation	2
Occasional cough or resistance to ventilator	3
Actively breathes against ventilator or coughs regularly	4
Fights ventilator, coughing or choking	5

Continued

Table 14.1 *Continued.*

Physical movement	
No movement	1
Occasional, slight movement	2
Frequent, slight movement	3
Vigorous movement limited to extremities	4
Vigorous movement including torso and head	5
Blood pressure (MAP) baseline	
Blood pressure below baseline	1
Blood pressure consistently at baseline	2
Infrequent elevations of 15% or more (1–3)	3
Frequent elevations of 15% or more (more than 3)	4
Sustained elevation of ≥15%	5
Heart rate baseline	
Heart rate below baseline	1
Heart rate consistently at baseline	2
Infrequent elevations of ≥15% above baseline (1–3) during observation period	3
Frequent elevations of ≥15% above baseline (more than 3)	4
Sustained elevation of ≥15%	5
Muscle tone	
Muscles totally relaxed; no muscle tone	1
Reduced muscle tone	2
Normal muscle tone	3
Increased muscle tone and flexion of fingers and toes	4
Extreme muscle rigidity and flexion of fingers and toes	5
Facial tension	
Facial muscles totally relaxed	1
Facial muscle tone normal; no facial muscle tension evident	2
Tension evident in some facial muscles	3
Tension evident throughout facial muscles	4
Facial muscles contorted and grimacing	5
Total score	

For children who are chemically paralysed, bispectral index scoring (BIS) (advanced skill) has been found to correlate well with the Comfort Score (Crain *et al.* 2002). The following BIS scores indicate levels of sedation:

- Very deep: <40
- Deep: 41–60
- Moderate: 61–80

- Light: >80
- Full consciousness: 95–100

(*Note here any other tools in your clinical unit:*)

For all children receiving sedation therapy check that the following is monitored (SIGN 2004) (basic skill):

- respiratory examination (see Chapter 2);
- cardiovascular examination (see Chapter 4);
- neurological monitoring: GCS scoring (see Chapter 7);
- intravenous access (see above);
- electrocardiogram (ECG) (see Chapter 5);
- oxygen therapy and pulse oximetry (see Chapter 3).

When there is prolonged or high dosage use of sedative drugs (Tobias 2000), check for (advanced skill):

- Tolerance: drug dose needs to be increased to maintain the same effect (due to down-regulation of receptors).
- Dependence: withdrawal symptoms may occur up to 3 weeks after stopping the drug and last for up to 6–8 weeks. Sedative drugs should be withdrawn slowly, alternative drugs introduced as required and the use of non-medicated therapy used where possible. Look for:
  o confusion, anxiety, agitation
  o muscle tremors
  o sweating
  o depression
  o dyskinetic mouth movements
  o toxic psychosis
  o convulsions
  o ataxia.

PAIN SCORING
(Basic skill)
Pain assessment should include a range of strategies (RCN 1999) and incorporate the use of:

- self-reporting (over 3 years of age)/parental assessment;
- behavioural measures;
- physiological measures.

Note that when:

- asking about pain, the caregiver must know what term the child uses for pain;
- selecting a pain assessment tool, it must be based on the child's age and cognitive ability (Franck *et al*. 2000);
- pain history is being taken, consider the following factors (Oakes 2001):
  - P (palliative and provocative factors): what makes the pain better? What makes the pain worse?
  - Q (quality): what does the pain feel like?
  - R (region and radiation): where is the pain? Where does it spread?
  - S (severity): how bad is the pain? On a score from 1–10, with 10 being the very worst, what number represents the pain (or use other scales, e.g. FACES – see below)?
  - T (timing): when did the pain start? How long has the pain been there? Is it constant or intermittent?
- there is a decreased conscious level, self-reporting becomes less viable;
- the child is critically ill and chemically paralysed, physiological parameters (see below) become the assessment tool.

Neonates and infants
Assess:

- babies cannot self-report pain but parents may be able to identify pain.
- hand twitching, jerking leg or head movements, frowning, eyes shut tight, mouth stretching vertically or on an angle, silent or weak cry, fisting, pulling knees up or spreading feet (Ramelet *et al*. 2006).
- increase or decrease in blood pressure and heart rate; respiratory distress (may need oxygen therapy).

Validated tools to assess pain include:

- NIPS (Neonatal Infant Pain Scale) (Lawrence *et al*. 1993) for neonates;

- LIDS (Liverpool Infant Distress Score) (Horgan & Choonara 1996) for infants;
- PIPP (Premature Infant Pain Profile) (Stevens *et al.* 1995) for premature infants (not validated).

(*List here other tools used in your clinical practice*:)

Young children
Assess:

- young children may be able to self-report pain and parents will be able to contribute;
- crying, moaning, wimpering, grimacing, frowning, quivering chin, clenched jaw, restlessness, drawing legs up, jerkiness, pulling ear, reluctance to move, quiet, rubbing specific region;
- increase in blood pressure and heart rate; respiratory distress (may need oxygen therapy or increasing oxygen therapy).

Validated tools to assess pain include:

- TIPPS (Toddler/Pre-School Post-Operative Pain Tool) (Tarbell *et al.* 1992) for 18 months to 5 years;
- CHEOPS (Children's Hospital of Eastern Ontario Pain Scale) (McGrath *et al.* 1985b) for 1 month to 3 years;
- FLACC (Face, Legs, Activity, Cry, Consolability) (McGrath *et al.* 1985b) for 3–7 years.

(*List here other tools used in your clinical practice*:)

Older children
Assess:

- can self-report pain;
- wimpering, moaning, crying, frowning, clenched jaw or hands, restlessness, drawing up legs, reluctance to move, quiet, rubbing specific region;
- increase in blood pressure and heart rate; respiratory distress (may need oxygen therapy or increasing oxygen therapy).

Validated tools to assess pain include:

- FACES (McGrath *et al.* 1985a) for 3–7 years;
- VAS (Visual Analogue Scales) (Scott & Huskisson 1979) for 3–7 years;
- OUCHER (Beyer 1984) for 3–7 years.

(*List here other tools used in your clinical practice*:)

Older child/young person
Assess:

- can self-report pain;
- frowning, restlessness, drawing up legs, quiet, rubbing specific region, reluctance to move;
- increase in blood pressure and heart rate; respiratory distress (may need oxygen therapy or increasing oxygen therapy).

Validated tools to assess pain include:

- APPT (Adolescent Pediatric Pain Tool) (Savedra *et al.* 1990) for 7 years and older;
- Ladder Scale (Beyer & Wells 1989) for young people.

(*List here other tools used in your clinical practice*:)

ENVIRONMENT CHECK
The impact of the environment on the acute/critically ill child is significant and includes sensory overload and deprivation, leading to interference with normal growth and development (including regression) as well as psychological problems. Bowlby (1960) suggests three stages of separation anxiety in infants and young children: protest, despair and denial. Table 14.2 outlines the impact of hospitalisation on children (basic skill).

Children frequently have interventions throughout the day and night (Al-Samsam & Cullen 2005). Toddlers are a particular challenge as they significantly develop physically, emotionally and intellectually through insatiable curiosity yet still cannot rationalise or verbalise effectively (Smith *et al.* 2003).

Table 14.2 Impact of hospitalisation.

Age	Impact of hospitalisation	Check that
Infant	Stress of light, noise and lack of caregiving activities: • jittery and agitated, raised pulse and BP, abnormal breathing pattern, hiccups or gagging, not tolerating feeds Separation from parents • initially protests but then stops loud crying; then may become unreactive to surroundings	Where possible, the same nurse is on each shift Control heat, noise and light Use comfort measures, e.g. toy, swaddling and supportive positioning Allow sucking and grasping Allow rest periods especially after procedures Encourage and support parental presence
Toddler	Development into autonomous beings is threatened; trying to explain procedures may not be effective (intellectually not developed) Stress of unfamiliar environment, temperature, noise, light – all frightening: • may cry fearfully; try to keep awake to watch what is happening despite exhaustion; may regress to an earlier stage of development Separation from parents is a major stress: • verbal protest and clinging, then may withdraw and become detached (toddler may think that he/she has done something wrong and that is why the parents have left)	Try to give some routine and ritual (preferably that which resembles toddler's normal day) to give back some control, but do not give a choice when there isn't one Encourage and support parents to stay with child; or have many reminders of the parents around the child Provide familiar toys, clothes, music, etc. Give lots of praise and reassurance that the hospital stay/illness is not child's fault Provide consistent nurses

Continued

Table 14.2 *Continued.*

Age	Impact of hospitalisation	Check that
Pre-schooler	Stress when child cannot accomplish things:	The child can help him-/herself whenever possible
	• may see being in hospital as being a punishment for something he/she has done wrong	Explain things in basic terms child can understand – do this just before the procedure, include the equipment and who is there to help
	• may have exaggerated fears as children are 'magical thinkers'	Have daily routines where possible
	Separation anxiety is less aggressive but still strong:	Provide therapeutic play and schooling
	• may refuse care or not communicate with others, leading to not eating and apathy	Encourage and support parents to stay with child; or have many reminders of the parents around the child
	• may regress to an earlier stage of development and/or take out fears on a toy or others	Provide consistent nurses
School age	A short stay tends to be less distressing:	Encourage and support parents to have maximum contact
	• may transfer frustrations into something else, e.g. anger/hit something	Encourage familiar things from home to be brought into hospital
	• still has a need for reliable contact with parents	Provide consistent nurses
	A longer stay may result in apprehensive behaviour and/ or regression to an earlier stage	Provide a routine similar to home as much as possible
		Encourage information from/contact with friends

	• nail biting, hair twirling • detachment with crying • tremors Intellectually more mature and so has less exaggerated fears and fantasises less • understands concrete explanations but may have a fear of injury to own body and loss of self-control	Encourage the child to say what is bothering him/her so that any unreasonable fears can be corrected Give praise and positive feedback
Young person	May impact on the transition from child to adult Older children tolerate illness least well as it interferes with their drive for independence Anxious about their physical appearance, their bodily function and fear of death • agitation may cause withdrawal or depression May feel depersonalised if can hear conversation about themselves Anxious about separation from friends (loss of social status) • may become uncooperative	Orientate to the ward Give full explanations Provide consistent nurses Provide liberal visiting by friends and family Ensure informed consent Set flexible limits and give choice within the ward Encourage self care Ensure participation in care planning Talk to and listen to the young person – get to know him/her as an individual

Assess for sensory overload and deprivation (basic skill):

- Noise: constant and frequent. Noise levels should not exceed 35 dB indoors and 30 dB in bedrooms (WHO 1999). The impact on the child includes:
- startling;
- digestive secretion reduction;
- hearing damage;
- increased heart rate, metabolism and oxygen consumption;
- sleep deprivation (see Table 14.3);
- headaches and fatigue;
- decreased growth hormones;
- increased pain and need for analgesia;
- release of stress hormones;
- interference with immune response and delay in wound healing;
- ITU (intensive treatment unit) psychosis.
- Light: excessive and constant (basic skill). The impact on the child includes:
  - confusion of day and night;
  - sleep deprivation (see Table 14.3).
- Unfamiliar tactile and olfactory stimulation/non-therapeutic touch: includes hospital food and smells, medicines, procedures.
- Pain and discomfort (basic skill): from procedures, interruption to family life.
- Lack of privacy (basic skill): the child is nursed in a large open unit or ward, aware of procedures and crises nearby, with strangers coming into the unit and being physically exposed to them and other children (Popovich 2003).
- Lack of normal beneficial stimulation (basic skill): familiar routines and rituals are removed, movement may be restricted and other people are now directing the child's behaviour; interferes with the child's coping mechanism; loss of control and power.

Table 14.3 Barriers to sleep and the effects of sleep deprivation (Scrimshaw *et al.* 1966; Phillipson *et al.* 1980; Chen & Tang 1989; Bonnet *et al.* 1991; Benca & Quintans 1997; Landis *et al.* 1997).

Barriers to sleep	Effects of sleep deprivation
Environment: • voices • telephones • pagers and bleepers • closing bins • use of equipment • footsteps • alarms • fluorescent lighting • temperature changes Physical: • invasive lines and tubes • discomfort from immobility • physiotherapy and suctioning • pain and discomfort from the underlying condition • physiological and psychological stress Medications: • adrenaline • noradrenaline • opioids (produce predominance in stage 1 non-REM sleep) • benzodiazepines (decreases REM sleep so prolongs SW sleep stages 3–4) Procedures and interventions: • emergency procedures and treatment • insertion of invasive lines • X-rays • nursing care • pressure area care • medical examinations	Diminished cell division and protein synthesis: • impairs growth and healing Decreases immune function: • increases risk of infection Increases oxygen consumption and carbon dioxide production: • irregular breathing • tissue hypoxia and acidosis • decreased level of consciousness • decreased respiratory muscle function (after 30 hours sleep loss) Negative nitrogen balance: • poor nutrition • feeding intolerance • tissue catabolism Impaired thermoregulation: • unable to maintain normal temperature Loss of stage 4 non-REM sleep: • muscle weakness • nausea • diarrhoea/constipation • headache • lack of co-ordination Psychological impact (after only 24–48 hours of REM sleep loss) can lead to psychosis (also known as 'ITU syndrome'): • apathy and withdrawal • restlessness, anxiety • jitteryness • irritability • inappropriate speech • tremors and shaking • rocking or head banging • anger • aggression • lack of orientation to time and place • hallucinations • picking at imaginary objects • feelings of persecution Drugs with a psychiatric impact: • opioids • inotropes • corticosteroids • antiarrhythmics

Assess for strategies to reduce noxious stimuli, maximise therapeutic touch and prevent psychological damage (basic skill):

- Family-centred care, including family at the bedside as often as possible, friends visiting as appropriate, cultural and spiritual activities;
- appropriate growth and development tools, e.g. toys, music, games, interaction, school activities, reassurance, swaddling and containment;
- promote familiar environment, e.g. own blankets, clothing, toys, photos of family and home;
- promote familiar routines wherever possible, e.g. bath time, teeth cleaning, radio, TV programmes;
- maintain privacy as much as possible: use curtains and appropriate clothing and covering;
- work with the family and child to select appropriate nutritional foodstuffs;
- pain and sedation scoring;
- decrease noise levels: quiet/sleep times are protected wherever possible; alarms and phones set at minimum safe level;
- day/night routine, including dimming lights whenever possible, clock visible, procedures completed during the day;
- age-appropriate communication and use of communication tools as and if possible, including adequate information and age-appropriate preparation for procedures; give choices where there is a choice.

SUMMARY

Caring for the sick child involves an holistic approach – a family-centred care approach. The child and family rely on the health care practitioner to act as advocate for the child's best practice in comfort and hygiene related to his or her developmental stage. Short visits to hospital may have a less detri-mental effect on growth and development. The health care practitioner must act to minimise these detrimental effects at all times.

REFERENCES

Al-Samsam, R.H. & Cullen, P. (2005) Sleep and adverse environmental factors in sedated mechanically ventilated pediatric intensive care patients. *Pediatric Critical Care Medicine*, **6** (5), 562–567.

Anderson, T. (2004) Cochrane made simple: topical umbilical cord care at birth. *The Practising Midwife*, **7** (10), 39–41.

Barnason, S., Graham, J. & Wild, M.C. (1998) Comparison of two endotracheal tube securement techniques on unplanned extubation, oral mucosa, and facial skin integrity. *Heart and Lung*, **27** (6), 409–417.

Benca, R.M. & Quintans, J. (1997) Sleep and host defenses: a review. *Sleep*, **20**, 1027–1037.

Bergstrom, N., Allman, R.M. & Alvarez, O.M. (1994) *Treatment of Pressure Ulcers*. Clinical Practice Guideline no. 15, AHCPR Pub. 95-0652. US Department of Health and Human Services, Public Health Service, Agency for Health Care Policy and Research, Rockville.

Beyer, J.E. (1984) *The Oucher: A User's Manual and Technical Report*. Judson Press, Evanston.

Beyer, J. & Wells, N. (1989) The assessment of pain in children. *Pediatric Clinics of North America*, **36**, 837–854.

Bickley, L.S. (2003) *Bates Guide to Physical Examination and History Taking*, 8th edn. Lippincott, Williams and Wilkins, Philadelphia, Chapters 6 and 17.

Bonnet, M.H., Berry, R.B. & Arand, D.L. (1991) Metabolism during normal, fragmented, and recovered sleep. *Journal of Applied Physiology*, **71**, 1112–1118.

Bowlby, J. (1960) Separation anxiety. *International Journal of Psychoanalysis*, **41** (2/3), 89–113.

Carnevale, F.A. & Razack, S. (2002) An item analysis of the comfort scale in a pediatric intensive care unit. *Pediatric Critical Care Medicine*, **3**, 177–180.

Chen, H. & Tang, Y. (1989) Sleep loss impairs inspiratory muscle endurance. *American Review of Respiratory Diseases*, **140**, 907–909.

Cortese, D., Capp, L. & McKinley, S. (1995) Moisture chamber versus lubrication for the prevention of corneal epithelial breakdown. *American Journal of Critical Care*, **4** (6), 425–428.

Crain, N., Slonim, A. & Pollack, M. (2002) Assessing sedation in the pediatric intensive care unit by using BIS and the Comfort scale. *Pediatric Critical Care Medicine*, **3**, 11–14.

Curley, M.A.Q., Quigley, S.M. & Lin, M. (2003a) Pressure ulcers in pediatric intensive care: incidence and associated factors. *Pediatric Critical Care Medicine*, **4** (3), 284–290.

Curley, M.A.Q., Razmus, I.S. & Marx, C. (2003b) Predicting pressure ulcer risk in pediatric patients: the Braden Q Scale. *Nursing Research*, **52**, 22–23.

Dore, S., Buchan, D., Coulas, S., *et al.* (1998) Alcohol versus natural drying for newborn cord care. *Journal of Obstetric, Gynaecologic and Neonatal Nursing*, **27**, 621–627

Doughty, D. (2004) Wound assessment: tips and techniques. *Advances in Skin and Wound Care*, **17** (7), 369–372.

Fairley, J.A. & Rasmussen, J.E. (1983) Comparison of stratum thickness in children and adults. *Journal of the American Academy of Dermatology*, **8**, 652–654.

Feber, T. (1995) Mouth care for patients receiving oral irradiation. *Professional Nurse*, **10** (10), 666–670.

Franck, L.S., Greenburg, C.S. & Stevens, B. (2000) Pain assessment in infants and young children. *Pediatric Clinics of North America*, **43** (3), 487–512.

Gaili, H. & Woodruff, G.H.A. (2002) Exogenous pseudomonas endophalmitis: a cause of lens enucleation. *Archives of Disease in Childhood, Fetal and Neonatal Education*, **86**, 204–206.

Geistlich (1993) *The New Concept in Wound Treatment Geistlich Geliperm Liquid Gel*. Geistlich Sons Ltd., Chester.

Gibson, F. & Nelson, W. (2000) Mouth care for children with cancer. *Paediatric Nursing*, **12** (1), 18–22.

Horgan, M. & Choonara, I. (1996) Measuring pain in neonates: an objective score. *Paediatric Nursing*, **8** (10), 24–27.

Infusion Nurses Society (INS) (2006) Infusion nursing standards of practice. *Journal of Infusion Nursing*, **29** (1S), S1–S92.

Jackson, A. (1998) Infection control: a battle in vein infusion phlebitis. *Nursing Times*, **94** (4), 68–71.

Kite, K. & Pearson, L. (1995) A rationale for mouth care: the integration of theory with practice. *Intensive and Critical Care Nursing*, **11**, 71–76.

Landis, C., Savage, M. & Lentz, M. (1997) Sleep deprivation alters body temperature dynamics to mild cooling and heating, not sweating threshold in women. *Sleep*, **21**, 101–108.

Lawrence, J., Alcock, D., McGrath, P., Kay, J., MacMurray, S.B. & Dulberg, C. (1993) The development of a tool to assess neonatal pain. *Neonatal Network*, **12**, 59–65.

Lund, C., Kuller, J., Lane, A., Lott, J.W. & Raines, D.A. (1999) Neonatal skin care: the scientific basis for practice. *Neonatal Network*, **18** (4), 15–25.

Lund, C., Kuller, J., Lane, A., Lott, J.W., Raines, D.A. & Thomas, K. (2001a) Neonatal skin care: evaluation of the AWHONN/NANN research-based practice project on knowledge and skin care practices. *Journal of Obstetric, Gynaecologic and Neonatal Nursing*, **30** (1), 30–40.

Lund, C., Osbourne, J., Kuller, J., Lane, A., Lott, J.W. & Raines, D.A. (2001b) Neonatal skin care: evaluation of the AWHONN/NANN research-based practice project on knowledge and skin care practices. *Journal of Obstetric, Gynecologic and Neonatal Nursing*, **30** (1), 41–51.

Madeya, M. (1996) Oral complications from cancer therapy: Part 2. Nursing implications for assessment and treatment. *Oncology Nursing Forum*, **23** (5), 808–819.

McGrath, P.A., Develoer, L.L. & Hearn, M.J. (1985a) Multidimensional pain assessment in children. *Advanced Pain Research Therapy*, **9**, 387–393.

McGrath, P.J., Johnstone, G., Goodman, J.T., Schillinger, J., Dunn, J. & Chapman, J. (1985b) CHEOPS: a behavioural scale for rating postoperative pain in children. In: Fields, H.L., *et al.* (eds) *Advances in Pain Research and Therapy*. Raven Press, New York.

McNeil, H.E. (2000) Biting back at poor oral hygiene. *Intensive and Critical Care Nursing*, **16**, 367–372.

National Institute for Health and Clinical Excellence (NICE) (2005) *The Prevention and Treatment of Pressure Ulcers*. Royal College of Nursing, London.

Oakes, L.L. (2001) Caring practices: providing comfort. In: Curley, M.A.Q. & Moloney-Harmon, P.A. (eds) *Critical Care Nursing of Infants and Children*, 2nd edn. W.B. Saunders, Philadelphia.

Phillipson, E.A., Bowes, G. & Sullivan, C.E. (1980) The influence of sleep fragmentation on arousal and ventilatory responses to respiratory stimuli. *Sleep*, **3**, 281–288.

Pickersgill, J. (1997) Taking the pressure off. *Paediatric Nursing*, **9** (8), 25–27.

Popovich, D.M. (2003) Preserving dignity in the young hospitalised child. *Nursing Forum*, **38** (2), 12–17.

Ramelet, A., Abu-Saud, H.H., Bulsara, M.K., Rees, N. & McDonald, S. (2006) Capturing postoperative pain responses in critically ill infants aged 0 to 9 months. *Pediatric Critical Care Medicine*, **7** (1), 19–26.

Ransier, A., Epstein, J.B., Lunn, R. & Spinelli, J. (1995) A combined analysis of a toothbrush, foam brush and a chlorhexidine-soaked foam brush in maintaining oral hygiene. *Cancer Nursing*, **18**, 393–396.

Royal College of Nursing (1999) *The Recognition and Assessment of Acute Pain in Children*. RCN, London.

Royal College of Nursing (2003a) *Standards for Infusion Device Therapy*. RCN, London.

Royal College of Nursing (2003b) *The Use of Pressure-Relieving Devices (Beds, Mattresses and Overlays) for the Prevention of Pressure Ulcers in Primary and Secondary Care*. RCN, London.

Rubenstein, J.S., Kabat, K., Shulman, S.T. & Yogev, R. (1992) Bacterial and fungal colonisation of endotracheal tubes in children: a prospective study. *Critical Care Medicine*, **20**, 1544–1549.

Savedra, M.C., Tesler, M.D., Holzemer, W.L., Wilke, D.J. & Ward, J.A. (1990) Testing a tool to assess postoperative pediatric and adolescent pain. In: Tyler, D.C. & Krane, E.J. (eds) *Advances in Pain Research Therapy*. Raven Press, New York.

Scott, J. & Huskisson, E.C. (1979) Graphic representation of pain. *Pain*, **2**, 175–184.

Scottish Intercollegiate Guidelines Network (SIGN) (2004) *Safe Sedation of Children Undergoing Diagnostic and Therapeutic Procedures*. www.show.scot.nhs.uk.

Scrimshaw, N.S., Habicht, J.P. & Pellet, P. (1966) Effects of sleep deprivation and reversal of diurnal activity on protein metabolism of young men. *American Journal of Clinical Nutrition*, **19**, 313–319.

Skewes, S.M. (1996) Skin care rituals that do more harm than good. *American Journal of Nursing*, **96** (10), 33–35.

Smith, P.K., Cowie, H. & Blades, M. (2003) *Understanding Children's Development*, 4th edn. Blackwell, Oxford.

Stevens, B.J., Johnston, C. & Grunau, R.V.E. (1995) Issues of assessment of pain and discomfort in neonates. *Journal of Obstetric, Gynaecological and Neonatal Nursing*, **24**, 849–855.

Suddaby, E.C., Barnett, S. & Facteau, L. (2005) Skin breakdown in acute pediatrics. *Pediatric Nursing*, **31** (2), 132–148.

Tarbell, S.E., Cohen, I.T. & Marsh, J.L. (1992) The Toddler–Preschooler Postoperative Pain Scale: an observational scale for measuring postoperative pain in children aged 1–5. Preliminary report. *Pain*, **50**, 273–280.

Tobias, J.D. (2000) Tolerance, withdrawal and physical dependency after long-term sedation in the paediatric intensive care unit. *Critical Care Medicine*, **28** (6), 2122–2132.

Tombes, M. & Galluci, B. (1993) The effects of hydrogen peroxide rinses on the normal oral mucosa. *Nursing Research*, **42** (6), 332–337.

Waterlow, J. (1997) Pressure sore risk assessment in children. *Paediatric Nursing*, **9** (6), 21–24.

Waterlow, J. (1998) Pressure sores in children: risk assessment. *Paediatric Nursing*, **10** (4), 22–23.

World Health Organisation (WHO) (1998) Care of the umbilical cord. http://www.who.int/reproductive-health/publications/MSM_98_4/index/html.

World Health Organisation (WHO) (1999) Noise guidelines. http://www.who.int/docstore/peh/noise/guidelines2.html.

Index

abdomen, 192–3
  auscultation, 193
  checking for ascites, 194–5
  palpation, 194
  percussion, 194
acid-base balance, 50–57
age groups, 1–2
anaesthetic/flow-inflating
    circuits, 36, 37
anal area, 199
APGAR scores, 4, 5
apnoea monitors/mattresses, 75
arterial blood gases (ABG), 45, 47
  assessing oxygenation, 49–50
  assessing the acid-base
    balance, 50–57
  assessment of puncture sites,
    47
  blood gas analysis machine,
    48–9
  sampling, 47–8
arterial catheters, 122–5
arteries, 96–7
ascites, 194–5
auscultation, 9–10
  abdomen, 193
  cardiovascular assessment, 89–
    95
  respiratory assessment, 24–9

bathing, 313–15
behaviour, 166, 168, 297–8
birth details, 4–5
bladder, 197–8
blood gas analysis machines,
    48–9

blood gas monitoring see
    respiratory monitoring
blood glucose, 231–2, 247–8
blood pH, 50–57
blood pressure, 82–5
  central venous pressure
    monitoring, 127–8
  fluid status, 235
  intra-arterial blood pressure
    monitoring, 122–4
  intracardiac haemodynamic
    monitoring, 129–32
body mass index (BMI), 208
body posture, 95
breath sounds, 17, 24, 27–8
  added/adventitious breath
    sounds, 28–9
  referred breath sounds, 28
bruising, 286–7

calorimetry, 214
capillary blood gas sampling, 60–
    61
capillary refill time (CRT), 98, 236
capnography, 63–6, 67
cardiac index, 114–15
cardiovascular assessment, 79
  anterior chest, 85–6
  auscultation, 89–95
  blood pressure, 82–5
  body posture, 95
  fluid status, 235
  heart sounds, 89–95
  history, 80
  jugular venous pressure (JVP),
    86–7

cardiovascular assessment, cont.
  normal and abnormal findings
    infants, 99
    young teenagers, 100
  oedema, 95
  palpation
    cardiac assessment, 88–9
    peripheral vascular
      assessment, 96–8
  pulse, 80–82
  vital signs, 80–85
cardiovascular monitoring
  arterial catheters, 122–5
  cardiac index, 114–15
  central lines, 125–9
  central venous pressure
    monitoring, 127–8
  electrocardiograph *see*
    electrocardiograph
  haemodynamic monitoring,
    121–2
  intra-arterial blood pressure
    monitoring, 122–4
  intracardiac haemodynamic
    monitoring, 129–32
  transducers, 115–21
catheter assessment, 245–6, 320–
    22
central catheters, 125–9
central venous pressure
    monitoring, 127–8
cerebral function analysis
    monitoring (CFAM),
    185–6
cerebral perfusion pressure
    (CPP), 181–2
chest deformities, 18
chest X-rays, 69–74
child ages, 1–2
clubbing, 19–20, 21
coma scoring, 168–9
  best motor reponse, 171–2
  best verbal or grimace
    response, 170–71
  eye opening, 169–70
comfort
  environmental check, 328–34

impact of hospitalisation, 328–
    31
pain scoring, 325–6
  neonates and infants, 326–7
  older children, 327–8
  young children, 327
  young persons, 328
sedation scoring, 322–5
sensory overload, 328, 332
separation anxiety, 328
skin integrity, 311–13
sleep deprivation, 333
continuous intra-arterial blood
    gas monitoring (CIBG),
    58–9
co-ordination, 150–51, 161, 162–3
  gait, 152–3
  point-to-point testing, 151–2
  rapid alternating movements,
    151
  reflexes, 143, 144–5, 153–5
coughs, 20–21
cranial nerves, 271–4, 275

deep tendon reflexes, 153–5, 160
dehydration, 232, 234, 235, 236,
    237–8
deprivation, 328, 332
developmental stages, 134–43
dietary requirements, 212
drug dosages, 210–11
drug infusions, 243–5
drug pharmacodynamics/
    pharmacokinetics, 300

ears
  hearing acuity, 263–4
  inspection and palpation, 263
  otoscope examination, 264–6
electrocardiograph (ECG), 103–
    106
  interpretation, 109–12
  normal electrocardiogram, 104
  right-side chest leads, 114
  six lead monitoring, 108, 112
  three lead monitoring, 106–108
  trouble-shooting, 114
  twelve lead monitoring, 112–14

electrolyte maintenance fluid
    solutions, 241–3
electrolytes
    fluid status *see* fluid status
    imbalance, 233
    normal levels and daily
        requirements, 231–2
endotracheal tubes (ETTs), 38,
    39
end-tidal carbon dioxide, 63–6,
    67
energy requirements, 212
    indirect calorimetry, 214
    predictive equations, 213
    stress factors, 212–13
environment check, 328–34
external ventricular drains
    (EVD), 182–4
extraocular eye movement
    (EOEM), 258–9
extravasation, 320, 322
eye care, 317–19
eyes, 234, 255–7
    extraocular eye movement
        (EOEM), 258–9
    ophthalmoscope examination,
        261–3
    visual acuity, 259–60
    visual fields, 261

facial expression, 15
facial features, 255
family history, 6–7
fluid administration
    drug infusions, 243–5
    electrolyte maintenance fluid
        solutions, 241–3
    hourly prescription rate, 240–
        41
    indwelling catheter
        assessment, 245–6
    normal daily maintenance
        fluid, 238
    normal hourly maintenance
        fluid, 239–40
    partial daily maintenance
        fluid, 239

fluid balance, 246–7
fluid status
    cardiac/vital signs, 235
    eyes, 234
    fontanelle, 233–4
    liver, 236
    mucous membranes, 234
    neurological state, 235
    oedema, 232–3
    renal, 236
    respiratory rate, 235–6
    skin turgor, 232
    vascular, 236
    weight, 236–8
fontanelle, 233–4, 251–3
fractures *see* musculoskeletal
    system
fremitus, 23

gait, 152–3, 284, 285
gastric tubes, 214–15
gastro-intestinal system
    abdomen *see* abdomen
    anal area, 199
    bladder, 197–8
    bleeding, 200, 201
    diarrhoea, 200, 201
    head and neck, 192
    history, 191–2
    liver, 196–7
    spleen, 195
    vomiting, 199–201
gastrostomy, 216–18
genitalia, 198–9
Glasgow Coma Score (GCS),
    168–9
    best motor response, 171–2
    best verbal or grimace
        response, 170–71
    eye opening, 169–70
glucose levels, 231–2, 247–8
Guillain-Barré syndrome, 160,
    164

haemodynamic monitoring, 121–
    2
    intracardiac, 129–32

haemodynamic monitoring, cont.
  see also cardiovascular
      monitoring
hair presentations, 256
head and neck, 192
  cranial nerves, 271–4, 275
  ears
    hearing acuity, 263–4
    inspection and palpation,
        263
    otoscope examination, 264–6
  eyes *see* eyes
  facial features, 255
  hair presentations, 256
  history, 250–51
  lymph glands, 270–71
  mouth and throat, 268–70
  nose
    inspection, 266
    internal examination, 267–8
    nare patency, 266–7
    sense of smell, 268
    sinuses, 267
  physical examination, 251–5
  techniques and findings for
      each age group, 276–8
  thyroid gland, 270
  trachea, 270
head box, 32, 35
head circumference, 208
hearing acuity, 263–4
heart sounds, 89–95
heat loss and gain, 298
  see also temperature monitoring
height, 208
history taking
  allergies, 6
  family history, 6–7
  identifying data, 2
  immunisations, 5
  medications, 6
  past medical history, 3–5
  presenting illness, 2–3
  previous illnesses, operations
      or injuries, 5
  psychosocial, 7
  review of body systems, 7–8

hospitalisation, 328–31
hygiene
  eye care, 317–19
  intravenous catheter
      assessment, 320–22
  mouth care, 315–17
  skin, 313–15
  umbilical care, 319–20
  wound assessment, 322
hyperthermia, 299–300
hyperventilation, 51
hypothermia, 300–301
hypoventilation, 51

infiltration, 320
injuries, 282
intra-arterial blood pressure
      monitoring, 122–4
intracardiac haemodynamic
      monitoring, 129–32
intracranial pressure (ICP), 178–
      81
intravenous catheter assessment,
      320–22

jugular venous bulb monitoring,
      184–5
jugular venous pressure (JVP),
      86–7

length, 208
limb palpation, 288–9
limping, 284, 285
liver, 94
  hepatomegaly, 236
  palpation, 196
  percussion, 196–7
  scratch test, 197
lymph glands, 270–71

malnutrition, 204–205
mental status, 175–6
midarm circumference, 210
motor system, 146–50, 161, 162
mouth, 268–70
  hygiene, 315–17
mucous membranes, 234

murmurs, 92, 93, 94, 95
muscle weakness, 146–50, 161,
    162
musculoskeletal system
  history taking, 280–81
    child with suspected non-
        accidental injury (NAI),
        282–3
    injured child, 281–2
    non-injured child, 282
  neurovascular assessment,
        291–4
  physical assessment, 283–4
    bruising, 286–7
    deformity, 286
    examination of the joint
        above and below, 284
    feel, 288–9
    limb palpation, 288–9
    look, 284–8
    movement, 289–91
    swelling, 284–6
    warmth of joint/limb, 289
    wounds, 287–8

nasal prongs/cannulae, 32, 34
nasogastric tubes, 214–15
nasojejunal tubes (NJT), 216, 217
naso-pharyngeal airway, 37, 38
neurological assessment
  co-ordination see co-ordination
  extinction, 158
  fluid status, 235
  infants, 158–60
  motor system, 146–50, 161, 162
  musculoskeletal system, 291–4
  normal growth and
      development, 134–43
  point localisation, 158
  pre-schoolers, 160–62
  reflexes, 143, 144–5, 153–5,
      159–60, 162, 163
  school-age children, 162–3
  sensory system, 155–6, 160,
      162
    light touch, 156–7
    pain and temperature, 156

    position (proprioception),
        157
    vibration, 157
  stereognosis, 158
  two-point discrimination, 158
  young persons, 163–5
neurological monitoring, 166, 167
  behaviour, 166, 168
  cerebral function analysis
      monitoring (CFAM), 185–6
  cerebral perfusion pressure
      (CPP), 181–2
  coma scoring, 168–9
    best motor response, 171–2
    best verbal or grimace
        response, 170–71
    eye opening, 169–70
  determining mental status,
      175–6
  external ventricular drains
      (EVD), 182–4
  intracranial pressure (ICP),
      178–81
  jugular venous bulb
      monitoring, 184–5
  limb movement, 172–3
  pupil size and reaction, 173–5
  seizures, 176–7
  significant events box, 175
  train-of-four (TOF) testing,
      186–7
  vital signs, 175
  neuromuscular blockade, 186–7
non-accidental injury (NAI),
      282–3
normal growth and
      development, 134–43
nose
  inspection, 266
  internal examination, 267–8
  nare patency, 266–7
  sense of smell, 268
  sinuses, 267
nutrition
  anthropometric measures, 210
  biochemical indices, 211–12
  delivery

nutrition, cont.
  gastrostomy, 216–18
  nasojejunal tubes (NJT), 216,
    217
  naso-/orogastric tubes
    (NGT/OGT), 214–15
  post-pyloric feeding, 216
electrolytes *see* electrolytes
energy requirements, 212
  indirect calorimetry, 214
  predictive equations, 213
  stress factors, 212–13
feed additives, 219
feed administration
  bolus feeding, 218
  changing feeding sets, 219
  choice of feed, 219
  continuous feeding, 218–19
malnutrition, 204–5
monitoring during feeding,
    220–21, 224–5
overfeeding, 223
tolerating feeds, 222–3
weight for calculating drug
    dosages, 210–11
nutritional clinical assessment,
    208–209
nutritional trigger assessment,
    205–207
  body mass index (BMI), 208
  head circumference, 208
  height, 208
  length, 208
  weight, 207–208
nystagmus, 258, 259

oedema, 95, 232–3
ophthalmoscope, 261–3
orogastric tubes, 214–15
oro-pharyngeal airway, 36, 37
otoscope, 264–6
oxygen masks, 31–2, 34
  with reservoir bag, 35–6
oxygen saturation monitors,
    44–5
oxygen tents, 32, 35

pain, 156
  scoring, 325–6
    neonates and infants, 326–7
    older children, 327–8
    young children, 327
    young persons, 328
palpation, 8, 263
  abdomen, 194
  cardiovascular assessment
    cardiac assessment, 88–9
    peripheral vascular
      assessment, 96–8
  limbs, 288–9
  liver, 196
  respiratory assessment, 22–3
  spleen, 195
peak expiratory flow, 66, 68
percussion, 9
  abdomen, 194
  liver, 196–7
  respiratory assessment, 23–4,
    25
  spleen, 195
percutaneous endoscopic
    gastrostomy (PEG), 216
peripheral vascular assessment,
    96–8
pharmacodynamics/
    pharmacokinetics, 300
phlebitis, 320, 321
physical examination, 8
  approaches, 10–11
  auscultation, 9–10
  documentation, 11
  inspection, 8
  palpation, 8
  percussion, 9
post-pyloric feeding, 216
posture, 95
precordium, 88–9
pregnancy details, 3–4
primitive reflexes, 143, 144–5
proprioception, 157
pulmonary artery, 130–31
pulse, 80–82, 96–7
pulse oximetry, 42–3

accuracy of SpO₂ readings, 46
oxygen saturation monitors, 44–5
probes and probe sites, 43–4
pulse pressure, 123
pulsus alternans, 85
pulsus paradoxus, 85, 97
pupil constriction, 173–5

radiation exposure, 71
radiographic views, 70
reflexes, 143, 144–5, 153–5, 159–60, 162, 163
respiratory assessment, 13, 29–30, 31, 32, 33
  accessory muscles, 18–19
  anaesthetic/flow-inflating circuits, 36, 37
  auscultation, 24–9
  chest expansion, 17–18
  chest recession, 19
  chest wall shape, 17
  clubbing, 19–20, 21
  colour, 15
  cough, 20–21
  endotracheal tube (ETT), 38, 39
  facial expression, 15
  fluid status, 235–6
  head box, 32, 35
  history, 13–14
  level of consciousness, 15
  nasal prongs or cannulae, 32, 34
  naso-pharyngeal airway, 37, 38
  oro-pharyngeal airway, 36, 37
  oxygen mask, 31–2, 34
    with reservoir bag, 35–6
  oxygen tent, 32, 35
  palpation, 22, 3
  percussion, 23–4, 25
  position, 14–15
  respiratory rate and rhythm, 15–17
  respiratory sounds, 17, 24, 27–8
    added/adventitious breath sounds, 28–9
    referred breath sounds, 28
  tracheostomy tube, 37, 38
  ventilator, 38, 40
respiratory monitoring
  apnoea monitors/mattresses, 75
  arterial blood gases (ABG), 45, 47
    assessing oxygenation, 49–50
    assessing the acid-base balance, 50–53
    assessment of puncture sites, 47
    blood gas analysis machine, 48–9
    sampling, 47–8
  capillary blood gas sampling, 60–61
  capnography, 63–6, 67
  chest X-rays, 69–74
  continuous intra-arterial blood gas monitoring (CIBG), 58–9
  end-tidal carbon dioxide, 63–6, 67
  peak expiratory flow, 66, 68
  pulse oximetry, 42–3
    accuracy of SpO₂ readings, 46
    oxygen saturation monitors, 44–5
    probes and probe sites, 43–4
    transcutaneous blood gas monitoring, 61–3
    venous blood gas sampling, 59–60

sedation scoring, 322–5
seizures, 176, 7
sensory overload, 328, 332
sensory system, 155–6, 160, 162
  light touch, 156–7
  pain and temperature, 156
  position (proprioception), 157
  vibration, 157
separation anxiety, 328

sinuses, 267
skin fold thickness, 210
skin hygiene, 313–15
skin integrity, 311–13
skin turgor, 232
sleep deprivation, 333
smell, 268
sphygmomanometer, 82–5
spleen, 195
stethoscope, 24
    see also auscultation
strabismus, 258
stress testing, 289–91
swelling, 284–6

temperature, 97–8
temperature monitoring
    drug pharmocodynamics and
        pharmacokinetics, 300
    hyperthermia, 299–300
    hypothermia, 300–301
    mechanisms of heat loss and
        gain, 298
    physical examination, 296–7
        behaviour, 297–8
        physiology, 298–9
    tools, 301–304
    warming/cooling methods,
        305–309
throat, 268–70

thyroid gland, 270
trachea, 270
tracheal deviation, 22
tracheostomy tubes, 37, 38
train-of-four (TOF) testing, 186–7
transcutaneous blood gas
        monitoring, 61–3
transducers, 115–21
triceps skin fold thickness, 210

umbilical care, 319–20
urine output, 236

venous blood gas sampling, 59–
        60
ventilators, 38, 40
visual acuity, 259–60
visual fields, 261
vital signs, 80–85, 175, 235
vomiting, 199–201

washing, 313–15
weight, 207–208
    calculating drug dosages, 210–
        11
    fluid status, 236–8
wounds, 287–8
    assessment, 322

X-rays, 69–74